Praise for *Separately Together*

"New paths present the traveler with uncertainty and a hint of danger. Without a map the journey can be perilous and painful. *Separately Together* offers a four-step roadmap for navigating one of the most challenging aspects of hospital administration. The book discusses key tactics such as pursuing a common language and creating respect by honoring distinctiveness. Simply stated, the book reinforces the mantra 'you get what you give.' With this guidebook in hand, the giving is less daunting and the path to healthy physician–executive relationships is navigable."
—Joseph R. Swedish, FACHE, President and CEO, Trinity Health

"*Separately Together* articulates a number of the counterintuitive truths necessary for physicians and hospital leaders to find common ground. The authors provide give a step-by-step process for to achieving a relationship that endures."
—J. Knox Singleton, President and CEO, Inova Health System

"The current debate over health reform has highlighted the absolute necessity of aligning hospitals and physicians—but the task is easier said than done. *Separately Together* is an excellent resource for healthcare executives, medical staff leaders, and their advisers who know that alignment must be done but need help doing it. Drawing on best practices from groups who have learned how to resolve similar conflicts, the book presents a balanced array of practical hints and proven techniques for mobilizing the stakeholders and moving them toward the benefits of collaboration."
—Jeffrey C. Bauer, PhD, Partner, ACS Healthcare Solutions

"*Separately Together* provides a refreshingly new perspective on the decades-old challenge of building collaboration between hospitals and physicians. It presents practical tools for managing the disconnect that often exists between physicians and hospital management. The authors supply specific strategies for aligning these groups in the quest for improving both clinical and financial outcomes."
—Errol L. Biggs, PhD, FACHE, Director, Graduate Programs in Health Administration, University of Colorado–Denver

"*Separately Together* is a valuable resource for new CEOs who have inherited a dysfunctional relationship with the medical staff. The book provides a road map for getting things back on track. The authors offer a unique way to solve the seemingly irreconcilable differences between physicians and healthcare executives."
—John Jeter, MD, President and CEO, Hays Medical Center

"The real difficulty in brokering physician–administrator understanding centers on getting the attention of the two groups and then finding the trusted leadership who can get to the early small wins. It is hard to get the real players together and keep them focused. The helpful tools described in *Separately Together* prompt folks to talk about commonalities instead of taking the typical positions."
—Donald A. Pocock, MD, FACP, CPE, Chief Medical Officer, Morton Plant Mease Health Care

"Hospital–physician relationships have been problematic since before Lyndon Johnson presided over the passage of Medicare. Over those years, many solutions have been proposed and tried by hospitals. *Separately Together* provides a timely and novel alternative to the traditional remedies. The book addresses healthcare executives and physician leaders who are dissatisfied with the status quo and the 'intractable righteousness' of the polar positions in this conflict. Based on careful review of the evidence from positive experiences, the authors propose a different process for sorting out the issues, separately emphasizing the worth and value of the participant groups, and reengaging for a common purpose. They lead the reader through that process with the help of case studies and numerous self-assessments and exercises. The book is a very positive and inventive new addition to the range of options available to hospital executives and physician leaders who are frustrated with current approaches and who are seeking a way to collaborate without capitulation."
—Michael Guthrie, MD, MBA, FACPE, Executive in Residence, Program in Health Administration, University of Colorado–Denver

"The premise of this book appears to be counterintuitive. The 'separate together' approach struck me as an oxymoron, but after reading this book, I found the logic compelling and the behavioral science supporting this approach irrefutable. The idea that physicians and executives must be confident and secure in their own respective value before a collaborative relationship can be developed provided me with one of those rare 'Aha!' moments. This book provides not only a creative approach to improving relationships but also interesting case studies and a prescriptive process for developing healthier relationships."
—James Shmerling, DHA, FACHE, President and CEO, The Children's Hospital

"The increasing level of conflict between physicians and hospital administrators is holding many organizations back from achieving breakthrough gains in quality, safety, and patient experiences. Authors O'Connor and Fiol outline an uncommon approach that transformational healthcare leaders can use to rewrite the future of their organizations. The authors provide a compelling case for performance improvement in organizations that apply the four-phase method described in the book. Case studies illustrate how the method can be applied at any hospital. This is an important book for leaders to read in anticipation of healthcare reform initiatives."
—John Lucas, MD, CEO, Cheyenne Regional Medical Center

"I enjoyed reading *Separately Together* and found it to be both timely and relevant given the issues hospitals and physicians are facing during this period of transformation. The self-assessment exercises were helpful and provided both a brief refresher on the key issues and an outline of the essential topics of discussion."
—Steven J. Summer, FACHE, President and CEO, Colorado Hospital Association

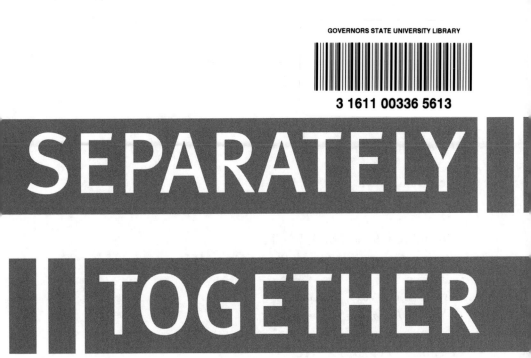

SEPARATELY

TOGETHER

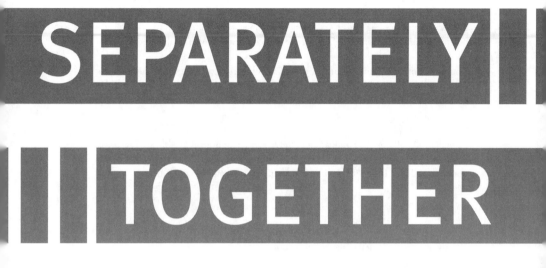

SEPARATELY

TOGETHER

A New Path to Healthy Hospital–Physician Relations

C. MARLENA FIOL • EDWARD J. O'CONNOR

HAP

ACHE Management Series

Your board, staff, or clients may also benefit from this book's insight. For more information on quantity discounts, contact the Health Administration Press Marketing Manager at (312) 424-9470.

14 13 12 11 10 09   5 4 3 2 1

Library of Congress Cataloging-in-Publication Data

Fiol, C. Marlena.
  Separately together : a new path to healthy hospital-physician relations / Marlena Fiol and Edward J. O'Connor.
    p. ; cm.
  Includes bibliographical references and index.
  ISBN 978-1-56793-337-6
  1. Hospital-physician relations. I. O'Connor, Edward J. (Edward Joseph), 1943- II. Title.
  [DNLM: 1. Hospital-Physician Relations. 2. Cooperative Behavior. WX 160 F517s 2009]
  RA971.9.F56 2009
  362.11068—dc22
                              2009014760

Acquisitions editor: Janet Davis; project manager: Dojna Shearer; book and cover designer: Scott Miller

Health Administration Press
A division of the Foundation of the
  American College of Healthcare Executives
1 North Franklin Street, Suite 1700
Chicago, IL 60606-3529
(312) 424-2800

For our children

Brad
Shannon
Shareen
Stefan

who have blessed us by so beautifully modeling the principles of
separate togetherness in our blended family.

Contents

Preface

IT IS NO secret that collaborative relationships between physicians and hospital administrators are critical for effective healthcare delivery. Neither is it a secret that, despite a proliferation of strategies, we have made little, if any, progress in our efforts to improve physician–hospital relations in the United States. Our current approaches to stemming conflicts are not working. Instead, conventional solutions provoke counterforces in a seemingly endless cycle. This book offers a new perspective on hospital–physician relations, based on evidence from social science research (e.g., Gaertner et al. 1999) and on practical experience from such diverse arenas as international diplomacy (e.g., Kelman 1998), corporate alliances (e.g., Hughes and Weiss 2007), and our own work with healthcare organizations: *To bring together groups locked in intractable conflicts, you must first pull them apart and strengthen them separately.* For the past several years, we have spoken to health system leaders and physicians about this perspective, and we have written about it (O'Connor, Fiol, and Guthrie 2006). The interest and enthusiasm we have encountered has led us to believe that a book is needed that outlines our approach and provides guidelines for its implementation.

This book describes the four phases of the PAR (Physician–Administrator Relations) Process for moving from intractable conflicts to enduring collaboration between hospital administrators and physicians:

1. Physicians and administrators must be *ready* to engage in a process of changing the relations between them.
2. The negative connections between the groups must be *disentangled* to reduce the intractability of the conflict.
3. The foundation for eventual collaboration must be laid by strengthening group members' *security* about their own group's distinctive value.[1]
4. The groups must learn to see the possibility of remaining secure in their own separate distinctiveness, even while aligning with the "other" around a common purpose.

Only after (a) readiness to begin has been developed, (b) the negative connections between hospitals and physician groups have been disentangled, (c) each group is secure in its unique value, and (d) each sees itself as a distinctive group and as part of the larger unit, is it possible to develop collaboration by promoting a common vision toward which both groups can work.

A common shortcut in healthcare is to attempt to "fix" conflicts by engaging the opposing parties in collaborative activities without first going through the earlier phases. A belief endures that with enough relationship-building activities (e.g., common goals, structural alliances), collaboration will result despite the intractability of the conflict. In fact, the books published in the last ten years that directly address physician–hospital relations generally begin with the premise that the conflicting groups should be brought *together* through change management and trust-building strategies (e.g., Annison and Wilford 1998; Atchison and Bujak 2001), conflict resolution and communication strategies (e.g., Cohn 2005; 2006), or increased medical staff involvement and integrative partnership arrangements (e.g., Holm 2000; 2004). Unfortunately, these strategies alone may not be enough (O'Connor, Fiol, and Guthrie 2006). They are likely to be useful only *after* the negative connections between the groups have been disentangled and people are secure about their group's unique and distinctive value (Fiol, Pratt, and O'Connor 2009).

This book is made up of three parts. In Part I, chapters 1 through 3 present the conflicts plaguing hospital–physician relations and the ways we have tried (largely unsuccessfully) to address them. Chapter 1 describes the unfortunate state of hospital–physician relations in the United States today and how it affects cost and quality. chapters 2 and 3 discuss traditional relationship-building approaches (e.g., creating a structural alliance or a common vision) and why they generally have not led to sustained healthy relations. In Part II, chapters 4 through 8 present our four-phase process for moving the groups from a state of intractable conflict to healthy and enduring collaboration. Chapter 4 introduces our overall approach (the PAR Process) and explains its social-psychological and practical underpinnings. The next four chapters describe each of the four phases of the PAR Process. Each chapter is organized in a similar fashion: We define the purpose of the phase, describe what it entails, and explain its importance. This is followed by a discussion of why it is likely to be resisted from all sides and a description of the process for moving through the resistance and achieving the intended outcomes. Finally, in Part III, Chapter 9 provides ten specific steps for beginning your journey to healthy hospital–physician relations and for sustaining the collaboration. It also lays out a number of pre- and post-process steps you must take to initiate the PAR Process and ensure its sustained success.

Each of the chapters in Parts I and II of this book ends with self-assessment questions for determining your organization's status with respect to the PAR Process. In addition, chapters 5 through 8 conclude with exercises to help you apply the steps of this process in your organization. The self-assessments and exercises closely mirror the material in each of the chapters and provide tools you can use to engage your people in the PAR Process. A running case describing events at Louis Martin Community Hospital (LMCH) is used throughout the book to illustrate the applicability of each phase and its links to the other phases. The case represents an amalgam of experiences we have had with numerous organizations; the organization and characters in the LMCH case carry fictitious names to ensure their anonymity.

This book is addressed to senior hospital executives and physician leaders who feel they can no longer win the game they are playing and who wish to remain and succeed where they are rather than jump ship and try again somewhere else. We are targeting the people on the clinical and administrative sides of the healthcare world who are working harder, longer, and faster and who feel it is just not working. We offer a new and promising solution.

NOTE

1. Neither physicians nor administrators are monolithic as a group, and many subspecialties/functions exist that fragment each of the groups into competing subgroups. The third phase of the PAR Process seeks to unify and strengthen both physicians and administrators as separate and distinctive groups, despite the many ways they have been fragmented in the past.

PART I

Physician–Hospital Conflicts and Traditional Approaches to Managing Them

CHAPTER 1

Hospital–Physician Relations Are at the Core of Healthcare Challenges

IN 2005, the United States spent $1.988 trillion, or $6,697 per person, on healthcare (Zhang 2007), twice as much as any other industrialized nation. Despite this investment, according to the Health Care Financial Management Association, the United States ranks lowest among developed nations in life expectancy and infant mortality (Shaman 2007). Healthcare costs are projected to rise from 16 percent of gross domestic product (GDP) in 2006 to 20 percent in 2015, and it appears unlikely that consumers will begin to get their money's worth for their healthcare dollars (Baicker 2006). As we write this in early 2009, the challenges facing U.S. healthcare continue to grow. Hospitals and health systems have experienced widespread layoffs, tanking investments, and uncertainties about their survival. Leo Brideau, president and CEO of Columbia St. Mary's, a Milwaukee-based three-hospital system, voiced the conclusion of many when he stated in late 2008, "This is just the beginning. I think it's going to get worse before it gets better" (Carlson 2008, 6).

A major barrier to successfully addressing the challenges our health systems face is the intractable cycle of conflict in which physicians and hospital administrators are often locked. Gary Filerman, chairman of the health systems administration department at Georgetown University, summarized the problem: "We're never going to achieve quality unless the adversarial nature comes out of teamwork" (Burda 2008, 26). In the words of world-renowned strategist Michael Porter (2008), "the *us-them* culture is a big part of the problem." These conflicts lie at the core of U.S. healthcare. When Jeff Goldsmith, a noted healthcare futurist, was asked what hospital executives need to do to navigate the environmental turbulence, the first item on his list was "reconciliation with the clinical staff" (Friedman 2003, 1). And according to a survey of hospital CEOs by the American College of Healthcare Executives (Carlson 2009), hospital–physician relationships ranked as one of the biggest worries, right after financial woes and care for the uninsured.

Relationships between hospital administrators and physicians are inherently ripe for conflict. Physicians view themselves as champions of patient care, while administrators see themselves as protectors of their hospitals (Hekman 2002). Though each group is highly interdependent and needs the other to survive and thrive, many physicians and administrators remain engaged in a destructive civil war. Increased pressures for quality outcomes, decreased reimbursements, more government regulations, and increasingly informed consumers combine to bring greater pressures to improve quality of care and reduce costs. Unfortunately, evidence suggests that U.S. health systems are doing poorly on both sets of outcomes (Baicker 2006). In fact, as we note later in this chapter, in many cases the increasing pressures for lower costs and higher quality outcomes further fuel the hospital–physician conflicts, leading to a vicious downward spiral.

We begin this chapter with an overview of the cost and quality challenges facing healthcare in the United States. We then describe the ongoing conflicts between hospitals and physicians as one of the major reasons that the healthcare industry has not been able to effectively address those challenges. We illustrate the deteriorating hospital–physician relations with a case study that demonstrates their insidious and damaging effects.

COSTS ARE HIGH AND RISING

As noted at the beginning of this chapter, the cost of healthcare in the United States is double that of any other industrialized country, and it is projected to continue to rise at a faster rate than the GDP. A 2006 survey conducted by Kelton Research on behalf of Edward Jones estimated that healthcare spending will reach nearly $3 trillion by 2009 and $4 trillion by 2015 (Ackermann 2006). And the rising cost of health insurance continues to drive a steady decline in employer-sponsored coverage and an increase in the number of uninsured people (Trapp 2007).

The problem of rising costs in healthcare is hardly new. Between 1945 and 1998 healthcare spending averaged a yearly 4.1 percent increase, compared with a 1.5 percent increase in GDP (Chernow, Hirth, and Cutler 2003). This ongoing upward trend is one of the factors weakening our economy. The United States must curb the rapidly increasing costs of healthcare. These costs are added to the cost of products and services, thereby crippling the nation's global competitiveness.

Of course, rising healthcare spending is not all bad, given the scientific advances in technology and drugs that account for some of it (Baicker 2006). For example, a PricewaterhouseCoopers' Health Research Institute study showed that drugs, medical devices, and advances in medicine accounted for 22 percent of the 13.7 percent healthcare premium cost increase from 2000 to 2001 (Kertesz 2004). In 2007, the same organization documented that the United States is the global leader in Nobel prizes for medicine and that four major recent healthcare innovations (MRI/CT, statins, CABG, and ACE inhibitors) were developed in the United States. Furthermore, the National Institutes of Health's research budget is $28 billion, compared to only $3.7 billion for all of the European Union (Shaman 2007).

Research and innovation are clearly benefiting from the healthcare dollars spent in the United States. But are customers and taxpayers getting valuable returns on that money? Are clinical and service quality improvements in line with the rising costs? As healthcare spending continues to grow more than two percentage points faster each year than the rest of the economy, it creates an unsustainable strain on private and healthcare budgets and exacerbates access problems for millions of Americans (Wilensky, Wolter, and Fischer 2007). The 2006 survey conducted for Edward Jones found that nearly a third of Americans said that not having enough money for healthcare is their biggest concern as they enter retirement (Ackermann 2006). As healthcare costs exert growing pressure on public and private budgets, it is essential that people get their money's worth for their healthcare dollars. As we note in the next section, evidence suggests that this is currently not the case.

QUALITY OUTCOMES ARE UNACCEPTABLE

At best, healthcare delivery in the United States is a wasteful process, involving too much work that does not add value to patient care, customer service, or the sustainability of the organization. For example, a study of 71 hospitals employing almost 75,000 people found that wasteful work consumed about 35 percent of employees' time (*Performance Improvement Advisor* 2003). And according to a 2005 report by researchers at Boston University, about 50 percent of healthcare spending is eaten up by waste, excessive prices, and fraud (Colliver 2005). Needless to say, 35 to 50 percent of spending going to waste increases costs without adding to clinical quality or service.

At worst, evidence indicates that our delivery system is falling far short of intended clinical outcomes. The following statistics published between 2003 and 2007 (Asch et al. 2006; Berwick 2003; Pavia 2003; Shaman 2007) illustrate why the CEO of Kaiser Permanente, George Halvorson, stated in late 2008, "Not only is American healthcare inefficient and wasteful, much of it is dangerous" (Connolly 2008).

- Despite the fact that U.S. healthcare spending was twice that of other industrialized countries, the United States ranked lowest in life expectancy and infant mortality.
- Only 55 percent of people received recommended care.
- The average hospital patient experienced at least one medical error daily.
- 50 percent of physicians did not adhere to documented and accepted clinical practice guidelines.
- 45 percent of general surgical patients were victims of inappropriate decisions.
- 2.6 percent of all hospital patients were injured by errors.
- Intensive care units (ICUs) averaged two errors per patient day.
- Serious medication errors occurred in 7 of 100 hospital admissions.
- More than 80,000 unnecessary hysterectomies and 500,000 unnecessary cesarean deliveries were performed in the United States each year.
- Only one in five elderly myocardial infarction survivors received proper medication to reduce the possibilities of reoccurrence.

Service outcomes are not much better. The average North American spends less than 30 minutes a year with a primary care physician. This is half as much time as patients in developed nations outside of North America (Fuhrmans 2008). Of course, less preventive care leads to greater use of emergency rooms. As emergency department patient volumes increase, patients are waiting longer to see a physician. According to Wilper and colleagues (2008), wait times increased 4.1 percent for all adult emergency department patients between 1997 and 2004.

By any reasonable standards, these outcomes are unacceptable. The U.S. healthcare system is a "tangled, highly fragmented web that wastes resources...leaving unaccountable gaps in care" (Fletcher 2005, 412). In a recent address, former president Bill Clinton (2008) referred to the United States as the world's "most diverse democracy." The rich cultural diversity of this country is one of our greatest assets, but it also presents challenges in adapting services to meet the needs of people of various backgrounds. The adaptive ability of our healthcare systems is directly proportional to the knowledge variety of service providers and the extent to which they can extricate themselves from the "tangled and highly fragmented web" to work together to meet the rising challenges.

THE NEGATIVE OUTCOMES ARE HITTING CLOSE TO HOME

Not only do negative cost and quality outcomes cause pain and suffering for consumers, they also leave their mark on healthcare professionals—on the clinical and administrative sides—who find themselves sinking deeper and deeper into a hole from which there seems to be no escape. Hospital administrators feel the stress of decreasing reimbursement, staff shortages, increasing pressures for patient quality and safety, changing technologies, increasingly empowered customers, an aging population, and increased competition (Atchison and Bujak 2001). They mourn for the time when they had a loyal medical staff and when their hospital was the center of the social structure for medicine. It is hardly surprising that the number of early retirements among healthcare CEOs has increased (Reilly 2004).

Physicians are not faring much better. They face decreasing autonomy, lower reimbursements, and increasing malpractice suits (Atchison and Bujak 2001). They also increasingly feel betrayed by a healthcare system that no longer gives them what they "signed up for": the respect, autonomy, recognition, and financial compensation they feel they deserve (LeTourneau 2004). The Center for Studying Health System Change found that physicians' inflation-adjusted income on average fell 7 percent between 1995 and 2003 (Evans 2007). Healthcare corporatization has resulted in a lack of trust, causing physicians to retire earlier and not to recommend careers in medicine to others (Anderson 2003). In one study, 56 percent of the 300 physicians surveyed said they would not choose a medical career if they had it to do over again (Greene 2000).

The following case study describes a real set of circumstances, even though we have renamed the hospital and the people involved to preserve their anonymity. We continue this story, based on experiences with a diversity of healthcare organizations, throughout the book. For the sake of continuity, we will refer to the exemplar organization throughout the book as Louis Martin Community Hospital.

Dissatisfied Managers and Physicians at Louis Martin Community Hospital

Years of noncommunication, miscommunication, and finger-pointing between physicians and administrators at Louis Martin Community Hospital had raised concerns among both groups about the costs of their inability to work together. As in many communities, anxiety over physician–administrator relations was near the top of the priority list. Leaders in both groups recognized that their inability to work together constructively kept them from making the necessary changes to improve quality and reduce costs.

The situation had intensified in recent months. To offset rising practice costs, a group of surgeons began to raise funds to open an ambulatory surgery center. Convinced that they could improve service, enhance quality, and reduce costs, they promoted their efforts as a contribution to the community. By expanding their control over medical decisions, physicians saw an opportunity to simultaneously expand their autonomy, improve patient outcomes, provide patients with better service, and improve their personal earnings.

Meanwhile, administrators—seeing one of their most profitable service lines migrating out the door—publicly accused the physicians of unfair competition and of undermining the hospital's ability to provide overall care. Angered by what they perceived as a lack of loyalty, a threat

---

(Continued on following page)

(Continued from previous page)

to their organizations, and a threat to long-term community health, they responded by threatening to remove the privileges of any physician who chose to compete with the hospital. This battle's clinical and financial costs to the community were clear to all. But neither side seemed able to disentangle itself from the long history of resentment and distrust and begin to reexamine alternatives together.

HOSPITAL–PHYSICIAN RELATIONS ARE AT THE CORE

The picture is bleak. As Figure 1.1 illustrates, rising costs and unacceptable outcomes feed each other and weaken morale to produce a negative spiral that can be difficult to break. Hospital–physician relations are at the core of this negative spiral, and no one seems to be winning. Hospital administrators and physicians alike are dissatisfied, and this seems to be worsening. As we noted, addressing the difficult relations between the groups ranks as a top priority for physicians (Press Ganey 2007) and hospitals (Carlson 2009). Both sides are bailing out because there seems to be no other option (Reilly 2004). If we do not clean up the mess in the center, no attention to costs or outcomes is likely to make a lasting difference.

The serious gaps in clinical/service quality and the widespread waste in the U.S. healthcare system directly reflect disjointed and poorly coordinated care systems, flawed care transitions, and failures of communication among caregivers and between clinicians and administrators (Fisher et al. 2006). Hospital–physician conflicts and competition lead to inefficiencies and waste in the form of continuous arguments that replay each side's view over and over. Hospitals and physicians increasingly compete for the same patient base using different business models (Weymier 2004), as in the case study about Louis Martin Community Hospital. From the hospital's perspective,

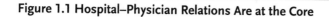

Figure 1.1 Hospital–Physician Relations Are at the Core

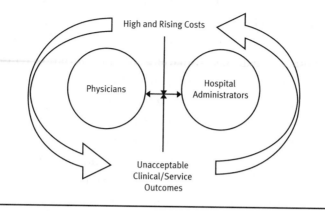

High and Rising Costs

Physicians

Hospital Administrators

Unacceptable Clinical/Service Outcomes

it was losing some of its most profitable lines of business, which resulted in a less financially favorable patient mix. In the long run, however, the hospital and the physicians run the risk of wasting valuable resources through excessive duplication of services, giving the community the impression that the healthcare providers are more concerned with their own financial interests than with providing quality, cost-effective patient care. The pressures resulting from the inevitable rising costs further fuel the conflict.

Competitive and distrustful hospital–physician relations have also negatively affected patient care and safety (Jeter 2003). Quality results depend not only on the skills and expertise of providers, but also on their relationships with one another (Clarke, Lerner, and Marella 2007). Errors occur when providers fail to coordinate their efforts. The competitive environment has led hospitals to avoid partnerships with their medical staff that could improve quality and safety (Dickey 2003). Hospital administrators contend that physician ownership of competing facilities can lead to unfair competition, as physician owners refer paying patients to their private facilities and send indigent and government-payer patients to the hospital (Semo 2003). And administrators are retaliating with their own form of control. For example, in early 2003, the governing board of

Community Memorial Hospital in Ventura, California, unilaterally imposed a code of conduct and conflict-of-interest policy on medical staff members that forbade any physician with a competing financial interest from serving as a medical staff officer or committee member, or voting on any medical staff matter. The administration refused to recognize the medical staff officers, including the chief of staff who had been elected by the medical staff, claiming that they had financial conflicts of interest with the hospital. A similar negative spiral was emerging in the case study. Naturally, the effectiveness of clinical care is compromised under these circumstances, and pressures resulting from service delivery failures exacerbate the conflicts.

Two decades of hospital–physician conflict and competition have made traditional relationships built on trust and loyalty increasingly difficult to maintain (Howard 2003). Things will only get worse if left unchecked. Younger people coming into the field are unlikely to develop the mutually supportive, long-term hospital–physician relationships that their predecessors did, since seeing many of those predecessors fired or forced into early retirement has led to widespread cynicism and distrust (Anderson 2003). In fact, a study of 21,672 physicians practicing at 224 U.S. hospitals in 2006 showed that younger physicians are notably less satisfied with their relationship with their hospital than are their older peers (Press Ganey 2007).

The issue is urgent. We know what the problems are, and we have been blaming external forces. For example, survey data from a recent study of hospital–physician relations in the United States and the United Kingdom found that a high proportion of hospital and physician leaders from both countries identified external factors, such as governmental budget cuts, pressure from third parties, and the turbulence of the policy environment, as important barriers to improving relations between hospitals and physician groups (Rundall 2004).

As long as the problems stay "out there," we will not be able to resolve them. Many traditional approaches are being desperately reinstituted. Both sides are exhorted to develop mutual trust, to return to hands-on relationships, and to explore partnership alternatives

(Howard 2003). The next two chapters describe common approaches to bringing the clinical and administrative sides of healthcare together and discuss reasons these approaches have seldom worked in the long run.

CHAPTER SUMMARY

This chapter provided an overview of the cost and quality challenges facing healthcare in the United States. Although relations between hospital administrators and physicians are one of many factors responsible for these challenges, we have argued that they are at the very core of the problem. This is because the ongoing conflict between the two groups prevents myriad other problems from being resolved.

SELF-ASSESSMENT EXERCISES

1. Gather information to determine whether physicians/administrators at your organization are aware of the financial challenges facing the healthcare industry. For example:

   What percentage of U.S. gross national product is spent on healthcare, and how does the United States rank relative to other countries?

   How fast is the cost of healthcare rising in the United States, and what implications does this have for:

   - Our citizens' ability to obtain access to healthcare services?
   - Our corporations' ability to compete internationally?

2. Gather information to determine whether physicians/administrators at your organization are aware of the clinical challenges facing the healthcare industry. For example:

   How does the United States rank in life expectancy relative to other industrialized nations?

   How does the United States rank in infant mortality relative to other industrialized nations?

3. Discuss the national quality outcomes described in this chapter with your senior leaders. Are these acceptable to you?

   Which, if any, of these outcomes describes the quality of care that patients using your services receive?

   What data have you collected to determine whether your performance is better or worse than these national averages?

How do physician–administrator relations at your organization affect your clinical outcomes and your ability to measure them effectively?

4. Do your leaders recognize that these issues necessitate urgent action to prevent others from controlling your destiny?

   Will your current physician–administrator relations allow you to respond to these urgent challenges effectively?

   What changes are necessary?

5. Do leaders regularly discuss hospital–physician relations as a major challenge to address? What new constructive recommendations have recently been put forward to improve these relations?

6. Assume that your organization continues on its present path with no major initiatives to change the current state of hospital–physician relations.

   Describe what physician–hospital relations will be like five years from now.

   What implications does your description have for your organization's financial and clinical outcomes?

   How will the hospital–physician relations you described affect the well-being of the people in your community five years from now?

   How will the hospital–physician relations you described affect the well-being of physicians and administrators at your hospital five years from now?

7. How are your leaders responding to decreased reimbursements, staff shortages, increased pressures for patient quality and

safety, changing technologies, increasingly empowered customers, the aging population, and increased competition in the healthcare industry?

Are you blaming others for these outcomes, or are physicians and administrators working together constructively to address these issues in your community? Are any leadership actions required to change this pattern so that the issues can be addressed more responsibly?

Do physicians and administrators at your organization recognize that distrustful, competitive relations negatively affect their ability to minimize costs and enhance patient care and safety?

What actions are required to increase physician and administrator commitment to minimizing costs and enhancing patient well-being?

CHAPTER 2

Structuring Our Way to Healthy Relations Hasn't Worked

INTRODUCTION

HISTORICALLY, HOSPITAL–PHYSICIAN relations in the United States were built on the basic premise that each party is separate and independent. Fee-for-service and cost-plus reimbursement systems meant little competition for healthcare dollars. Physicians could make decisions as they saw fit to benefit individual patients, and the community hospital was a center for medical technologies and a responsible and able social institution that could pass on extra costs in a cost-plus system. Hospitals and physicians coexisted in harmony but remained largely independent of one another. If we call the goals and the reason for existence of each their "dreams" and the structures in which they resided their "beds," one might say that hospitals and physicians in the early 1900s had different dreams and inhabited different beds.

Major institutional changes in the mid-1900s transformed hospitals from workshops for local physicians into powerful economic systems, and new business models for healthcare delivery gained legitimacy. Changing reimbursement systems and increased competition for healthcare dollars beginning in the 1970s exacerbated this shift. The introduction of managed care and the growing legitimacy of administrators and their business models throughout the 1980s and 1990s led to a perceived need for economic and legal strategies to align physicians with hospitals to gain market power in a fiercely competitive managed care environment. Structural and contractual integration quickly became an accepted method for managing hospital–physician relations in a world in which competition is more common than collaboration. The underlying logic seemed to be that if you put hospitals and physicians in the same bed, they will begin to share the same dream, and alignment will follow.

This chapter provides a broad overview of structural attempts to align hospitals and physicians and a rationale for why these attempts have generally failed to align the groups around a shared dream. Our aim is not to provide a comprehensive account of the many structural forms of hospital–physician integration that have emerged in the past decades, since this has been covered elsewhere in great detail (Holm 2000).

ONE BED

As noted in Chapter 1, decreased reimbursements; increased pressures from government regulations; increased demand for improved quality, safety, and service outcomes; and demands for lower costs combine to make physicians and hospitals more accountable. Health plans that had previously simply paid for physician services became active managers of the premium dollar, often determining the appropriateness of the services physicians and hospitals were providing.

Given that physicians control the majority of medical costs within hospitals, it is not surprising that hospitals felt the need to align with them to succeed in the changing environment. The 1980s and 1990s witnessed a push for hospital–physician structural integration to combat the growing competition for decreasing reimbursement and to maintain market share. This integration took many forms, but vertical integration was thought to be one of the most sustainable models. The belief was that membership in a vertically integrated group would result in trust, cooperation, and improved quality of care (Budetti et al. 2002).

One common way to vertically integrate physicians into hospitals was through direct ownership of physician practices. If hospitals owned physician groups the theory was that they would be aligned through shared goals and objectives. Hospitals' rationales included ensured referrals, clout with managed care, and a defense against those practices being acquired by other hospital systems. Perceived benefits to physicians included market clout, not having to deal directly with managed care, and access to capital. Such integrated systems were expected to increase efficiency in patient care by allowing hospitals and physicians to combine their operations. The new systems would create treatment guidelines leading to better patient care. In addition, it was believed that integration would result in cost savings, increases in services offered, risk sharing, and enhanced market positioning. As of this writing in 2009, hospitals are still buying up physician practices.

For the most part, these vertically integrated delivery systems have failed to produce the intended results. A study published by the Medical Group Management Association in 2008 found that hospitals lost, on average, $67,000 per physician per year in their acquired practices in 2006, up from a loss of $58,000 in 2004 (Medical Group Management Association 2008).

The failed attempts to align with physicians through structural integration have intensified the already heated conflicts between physicians and hospital administrators. Physicians have become increasingly frustrated and angry. As one physician put it, "It's just no fun being a doctor anymore." And according to another physician's wife, "My spouse's judgment is constantly questioned by nameless and faceless corporate minions armed with the rule books" (Bottles 2000, 44).

Physicians have retaliated by demanding pay from hospitals for clinical or managerial roles or insisting on exclusive service arrangements, both designed to tap into the hospital's income stream. And they have begun competing with hospitals by offering medical options in niche markets, such as specialty hospitals, diagnostic imaging facilities, and ambulatory surgery centers (Strode 2004).

Of course, such actions have simply brought about counter-retaliations from hospitals, further straining the relationships. If physicians began a new venture, they could expect pushback from disgruntled hospital administrators, including the possibility of withheld credentialing or litigation (which hospitals generally have more resources to carry out). Alternatively, hospitals might simply choose to get rid of a physician who joins a local outpatient center (Cohn et al. 2005).

In sum, unrealistic expectations about throwing such diverse groups as physicians and hospitals into the same bed have frustrated attempts at full integration. The pressing issue for hospitals has continued to be protection of market share and clout, and they have needed alignment with physicians in order to gain this advantage. In the latter part of the twentieth century, the focus turned to accomplishing this without the large financial losses that usually result from complete vertical integration. Would it help to share only a part of the structural bed? In other words, would partial integration deliver the benefits of alignment, and would it be cost effective?

PARTIALLY SHARING A BED

Strategic alliances became popular in the 1990s as an alternative to fully integrated systems. The goal was still to align physicians and hospitals to help control an increasingly hostile environment. Strategic alliances consist of two or more organizations that contractually pool resources to achieve a long-term strategic purpose that is not possible for a single organization (Judge and Ryman 2001).

Alliances quickly became a fad in the United States. In a 1997 nationwide survey of healthcare executives, more than two-thirds of the respondents indicated that they were engaged in one or more strategic alliances (Judge and Ryman 2001). Many of these were new: 33 percent of hospitals, 42 percent of managed care facilities, and 23 percent of physician group practices indicated that they had only recently entered into strategic alliances. Craig Holm (2000), in his book titled *Next-Generation Physician–Health System Partnerships*, noted that, according to a survey of health system CEOs, the most frequently employed partially integrated physician-hospital models in the 1990s were physician–hospital organizations (PHOs) and management service organizations (MSOs). In a 1995 American Hospital Association (AHA) survey on physician–hospital organization arrangements (Dynan, Bazzoli, and Burns 1998), approximately 1,300 hospitals reported such arrangements either directly or through a system/network affiliation.

PHOs are loosely coupled structures that divide the economic risks between the physicians and hospitals only for the specific projects and activities of the PHO. However, they typically have few managed care contracts and involve little capital investment by physicians, so there is little risk sharing between the two parties. Physicians retain ownership of their practices and can choose whether or not to engage in the joint-venture projects of the PHO.

MSOs, which commonly include service organizations from which physicians can purchase support services, may or may not have hospital ownership. For example, a hospital may own and operate a surgery center. Physicians could be given the opportunity to purchase equity in the service organization that is responsible for managing the center. While the MSO would be jointly owned by the hospital and physicians, the physicians could own a majority and appoint a majority of its board. The MSO would then enter into a management contract with the surgery center, giving physicians control of day-to-day matters.

As in the case of fully integrated structures, it was thought that such alliances would clinically and financially benefit the hospital, physicians, and patients. The community would benefit from the increase in services and good clinical outcomes. Physicians would benefit from increased revenue, increased efficiency, and greater control over operational processes affecting patient care. Hospitals would benefit from the increase in revenue if physicians agreed to not invest elsewhere.

Such alliances were also expected to minimize debates over technology expenditures (Broermann 2003). The reasoning was as follows: When the doctors are all engaged as partners in every aspect of the business, they are more apt to evaluate the expenditures critically and say, "Well, we really don't need it because the utilization or incremental efficacy would be minimal."

While the most frequently employed partially integrated physician–hospital models in the 1990s were MSOs and PHOs, evidence suggests that they were also the least effective (Holm 2000), and they soon began to look less appealing. According to the AHA, for example, 27.6 percent of hospitals had PHOs in 1994; this percentage grew to 33.2 percent in 1996 and then declined to 26.4 percent by 2000 (Bazzoli et al. 2004).

The problems in these alliances sometimes surface even before the partnership is consummated. For example, St. Catherine's Hospital and Kenosha Medical Center in Kenosha, Wisconsin, spent three years negotiating a partnership that could have saved up to $44 million over five years. However, constant conflict and trust issues kept the plans from materializing. St. Catherine's wanted full control over the venture, while Kenosha Medical Center felt that the new board of directors should have the control. In the end, they just called it quits (Judge and Ryman 2001).

Similarly, in 1992, the CEO of Ashtabula County Medical Center in northeast Ohio began negotiations to create a strategic alliance with 14 local physicians. Each side took a negative, adversarial approach from the beginning. They hired separate lawyers and picked their own terms with which to begin the alliance, which resulted in a failure to move forward. As one of the participants later noted, "We staked out our position and then sat down and tried to reconcile our differences. This approach immediately turned adversarial and nothing materialized" (Judge and Ryman 2001, 76).

The rush to partially integrate in the 1990s suffered a similar fate to that of the rush to fully integrate in the 1980s and early 1990s. It became increasingly clear that it matters little whether the structures are partially or fully integrated. Neither apparently results in aligning the dreams of hospitals and physicians.

WHY HAVE STRUCTURAL APPROACHES BEEN SO POPULAR?

It is not surprising that structural/contractual approaches were popular in the 1980s and 1990s. They potentially offered a relatively easy way to align the dreams of physicians and hospital administrators. The logic went something like this: Bring the warring parties together within the same legal/physical structure, and alignment will follow; put them in the same bed, and they will share the same dream. The idea was similar to that often used to justify bringing conflicting ethnic groups together: Structural integration would lead to mutual understanding and a greater awareness of the similar values and attitudes of the "other" (Cook 1984). This approach sought to reduce the ignorance caused by prejudice to enhance cooperation and coordination.

Not only did structural models appear to represent an easy fix for the problems of hospital–physician relations in the 1980s and 1990s, they also seemed like a safe bet, because so many hospitals and health systems around the country were doing the same thing. There is great safety—albeit illusory safety—in numbers. If two-thirds of all U.S. hospitals are involved in some sort of strategic alliance (usually PHOs or MSOs) with their physicians, it must be the most cost-effective and least risky form of aligning with them, right? Afraid of being left on the sidelines, other providers scrambled to follow suit.

This type of thinking drives the herd behaviors that are so prevalent in healthcare in the United States. It reminds us of the story of how we finally got rid of gnats on our houseplants at home:

Gnats had made our houseplants their home. A call to a plant doctor revealed an interesting strategy for getting rid of them: Put ¼ inch of a nasty-smelling whiskey, preferably white lightning, in a glass and set it next to the plants. Gnats love the stuff and will dive into it in droves and kill themselves. (O'Connor and Fiol 2002, 22)

Hospitals and group practices have been diving into structural white lightning of various kinds. Herd behaviors have been rampant. The widespread adoption of an innovation—be it an idea, a technique, a technology, or a product—when its benefits are unproven is common. Full and partial structural integration, intended to align hospitals and physicians, is one of the most dominant healthcare herd behaviors of the past two decades, despite a lack of evidence as to its real value (Coddington et al. 2000). While exceptions exist, many integration efforts have produced minimal value for the organizations involved (Colon, Gupta, and Mango 1999; Hoskisson and Hitt 1994; Jaklevic 2001), and some have killed participation as surely as white lightning kills gnats.

Lee Kaiser (2000), an eminent healthcare futurist, noted that "health care providers are 'me too' folks. They wait for someone else to do something first and then they rush to copy it." These behaviors are not hard to understand. Following the herd requires less of the hard work associated with thoughtful leadership. In the words of Bertrand Russell, "Many people would sooner die than think; in fact, they do so." Mindlessly copying others also minimizes personal risk by providing a ready justification for less-than-successful choices.

Case Study: Herd Behavior at Louis Martin Community Hospital
As CEO at Louis Martin Community Hospital, Mr. Joe Mosher was faced with mounting challenges. Housing prices in the community had tripled. People who had supported the community hospital for 80 years were moving on as factories in the area closed. Newcomers moving into the

---

(Continued on following page)

(Continued from previous page)

community seemed willing to drive 10 or even 30 miles to receive care from one of the multiple competitors.

Competition had grown fiercer. Physician referrals were not what they used to be, and Mr. Mosher knew that action needed to be taken to protect the long-term financial viability of the hospital.

To make matters worse, surveys of local residents suggested that many believed that LMCH's service was slow and that the clinical outcomes were questionable. Equally disturbing, the independent medical staff was openly critical when publicly discussing Mr. Mosher's administrative team, and there were rumors that a group of physicians was raising funds for a competing surgery center. The hospital's census numbers were dropping, and revenues and limited resources were drying out. Mr. Mosher needed to make significant choices while he still could.

As he looked at the solutions other hospitals were pursuing, he saw three options. Two of these (cost cutting through reduced services and selling to a larger system) would deprive the community of its control over a full range of services provided by LMCH. The currently popular option of forming a legal/economic alliance with physicians for the obvious benefit of all involved seemed far more palatable. After all, when he brought them all together in his organization, they would know each other better and would share a common commitment to market dominance, and performance would have to improve. Given how many of these alliances were being formed throughout the country, they *must* be the right answer.

Herd behaviors are hard to curb. Examples of structural failures are widespread and include PHOs, MSOs, physician employment models, and acquisition or management of physician practices by for-profit or not-for-profit organizations. All of these approaches come from the realms of structure, governance, and economics, and many have grown into "distressed marriages" possibly headed toward divorce (or already divorced). Evidence has shown that creating these organizational structures in no way guarantees alignment between hospitals and physicians (Holm 2000). A 1995 AHA survey found differences in the degree of integration achieved across the organizational models, but these differences had little to do with the structural form of the venture. This finding is significant, because it points to the fallacy of believing that structural or contractual integration is synonymous with coordination and alignment (Dynan, Bazzoli, and Burns 1998). Even with the majority of evidence showing negative results on investment return, some healthcare organizations continue to purchase physician practices (Epperson and Barakat 2006). And physicians continue to allow such purchases to gain financial protection from the hospitals or large systems, even though the alliance is not necessarily a good fit.

Healthcare is certainly not unique in its search for easy structural fixes to intractable conflicts. We see a similar pattern in attempts to address racial discrimination in the U.S. school system. In many school settings across the country, interracial, interethnic, and other intercultural tensions have been major impediments to improving student achievement, social behavior, and attitudes. Large-scale structural efforts, ranging from court-mandated school desegregation to implementation of multicultural programs aimed at bringing the different groups together, have been undertaken to address intercultural inequities and tensions. Despite these efforts, the intergroup strife continues to be a major concern of educators, students, parents, and the public (Cotton 2008); structural desegregation did not have the intended positive effect on achievement scores for students being bused (Sheehan and Marcus 1978); students continued to select their friends on the basis of likeness of race rather than likeness of mode of transportation (Wolf and Simon 1975); and there was significant "white flight" in reaction to busing (Lord and Catau 1976). These results point to the ineffectiveness of structural solutions for solving intergroup tensions among multiethnic students. (Research shows that in some cases bringing culturally different students into direct contact did appear to have a positive effect, but not simply because they were in contact. Rather, those successes were the result of carefully planned group learning activities performed under the right conditions [Cotton 2008].) In the ethnonational arena, too, we can see the temptation to integrate conflicting factions by physically colocating them. The ensuing violence in countries such as Rwanda and former Yugoslavia is a key example of the dismal failure of this approach (Kaufman 1996).

WHY HAVE STRUCTURAL APPROACHES FAILED?

Structural approaches to intractable intergroup conflicts appear to be an easy fix, and their popularity makes them seem less risky than other options, but they have generally failed to solve the problem. In some settings, attitudes and interactions have actually worsened (Cotton 2008). As one expert in the education field put it, "Integration does not just occur naturally as a result of merely placing students together in the same school setting" (Robert 1982, 3). Promoting contact has been shown to cause more harm than good, especially when the conflicting groups are brought together physically and given a task but not the tools to complete it successfully. Under these conditions, participants are likely to blame those who differ from themselves—in race, gender, ability, etc.—for the failure. Does this sound familiar?

It is not surprising that structural approaches to improved relations between conflicting groups (hospital–physician or multiethnic) have generally not led to the desired results and have often driven an even greater wedge between the parties. Placing people with a long history of animosity, distrust, and misunderstanding in closer physical proximity may simply allow them to fight more easily. When did more interaction with someone you dislike and feel little in common with ever lead you to change your beliefs about that person? Though it is surely true that more information about the other becomes available as a result of structural or physical proximity, the new information is not likely to alter ignorance or prejudice. We all tend to filter new information to conform to our existing beliefs (Northrup 1989). Therefore, in situations tainted by conflict between differing beliefs, any new information gained through structural integration is likely to be filtered in a selective way that simply provides further support for the negative stereotypes.

Stereotypes abound in healthcare, because physicians and administrators come from fundamentally different cultures. Administrators come from what is referred to as a "collective" culture (Atchison and Bujak 2001), which embraces the organization's values, mission, and vision. People in collective cultures like to work in groups, they generally avoid conflict, and they are relatively unlikely to take risks. By contrast, physicians come from what is referred to as an "expert" culture (Atchison and Bujak 2001), driven by the need for rapid decision making, autonomy, and individualistic behavior. People in these cultures have been inculcated with these norms and beliefs from a young age. Medical students learn that success is gained from individual achievements and accountability, while students of administration are taught the importance of long-term planning and delegation of responsibilities. These differences do not disappear simply because the groups become structurally bound to one another. In fact, if such groups are colocated, the differences tend to collide in even more dysfunctional ways, leading to further stereotyping and blaming. So despite allowing conflicting groups to gain more information about one another, structurally integrated healthcare settings maintain and even exaggerate existing stereotypes, until managing the partnerships and collaborating become impossible (Holm 2000).

CHAPTER SUMMARY

Relations between hospitals and physicians have continued to worsen during the past few decades, even while the structural integrative attempts were at their peak. Closer interactions within the same structural bed seem to increase rather than decrease costs, as they increase rather than decrease conflicts among physicians and hospital administrators. The battles have heated up as the conflicting parties have been thrown into the same bed, and this has certainly not led to following the same dream. The next chapter describes attempts to align physicians and administrators by focusing more directly on sharing a common dream.

SELF-ASSESSMENT EXERCISES

1. Clarify with your leadership team your business model and the assumptions that underlie it.

    What competitive advantage does your relationship with physicians/administrators provide in successfully implementing this model?

    Are your assumptions based on seeing physicians/administrators as competitors or as collaborators?

    What signals do you consistently provide that clarify for the 'other' your expectations about the relationship and how they should interact with you?

2. Collect the following information from physicians and administrators in your community:

    What percentage of them is currently optimistic about the likelihood that being part of the same organization leads to better understanding and mutual cooperation?

    What inducements would entice the 'other' into the same structural bed as you, and are they likely to lead to loyalty as well as exceptional clinical and financial results?

    What implications does this information have for the physician–hospital relations strategy you should pursue in the future?

3. List the primary fundamental values and behavior patterns of the physicians and administrators you know.

    What significant differences do you observe?

    What challenges are these observed differences likely to create if you bring the two groups together in the same organization?

Can these differences and the resulting challenges be realistically minimized to produce a successful venture?

4. To what degree has your organization participated in various healthcare structural fads, including mergers, PHOs, and MSOs?

How do this history and its results affect the way you currently think about your relationship with physicians (administrators)?

Is it appropriate to base your future interaction patterns upon this history, or are more constructive strategies currently available? If so, what are they?

5. What is your experience of being forced into close physical proximity with other people who have competing values/moralities/goals?

Has this experience led to a better understanding of and a positive working relationship with them?

What have you learned that is useful about making such relationships work?

How is this learning relevant to improving physician–administrator relations in your organization?

CHAPTER 3

Visioning Our Way to Healthy Relations Hasn't Worked

ATTEMPTS AT STRUCTURAL integration of hospitals and physicians have largely failed to align their interests and create a sense of joint destiny. Attempts at more direct integration have been made by focusing on aligning participants' values and beliefs rather than on structural alignment techniques. This represents a shift of focus from ownership to relationship and from structure to process. We refer to this approach as promoting a common vision or dream among the groups, whether or not they share the same structural bed.

Before examining the various attempts to align hospital administrators and physicians around a common dream, it is important to remember the fundamental differences that have created a chasm between the dreams each group holds today. As we noted at the end of Chapter 2, the conflicting worldviews are a result of a long history of differences in education and experiences. In fact, they started long before the groups began to clash in their healthcare work (Atchison and Bujak 2001). Physicians are trained in biomedical sciences and learn in school to work independently, not in teams. Medical school does not teach many team skills; instead, it breeds the philosophy that physicians need to think on their own and take responsibility for their own actions (Shortell 1991). By contrast, hospital administrators are educated in social and management sciences that emphasize the values of delegation and working in groups.

As a result, hospital administrators are drawn to a *collective* culture that embraces the organization's values, purpose, and vision (Atchison and Bujak 2001). Collective cultures are made up of people who prefer to work in groups, who avoid conflict, and who seldom take risks. By contrast, physicians are part of an *expert* culture, also found in engineering firms, architectural firms, and multispecialty law firms, among others. This culture is driven by individualistic behaviors that are motivated by autonomy and self-reliance.

This chapter provides an overview of attempts to integrate hospitals and physicians in the face of these cultural differences, by promoting a common dream that is based on a foundation of trust and open communication. We discuss why this approach has been so popular, and we conclude the chapter with a rationale for why it has fared no better than structural approaches for developing hospital–physician alignment.

THE UNDENIABLE CASE FOR SHARING A COMMON DREAM

Undeniably, sharing a dream that is based on a foundation of mutual respect, trust, and open communication improves relations between conflicting groups. In fact, one study of medical partnerships suggested that if a common direction was derived, conflicts among the partners could be reduced by 60 to 70 percent (Finger 2000).

Industries that have improved relationships through trust-building processes and the development of a common vision include pharmaceuticals, aerospace, and information technology. In their often-cited book, *Built to Last*, Collins and Porras (1994) present evidence that organizations driven by common values, purpose, vision, and goals outperformed the general stock market 15 to 1 over a 50-year period. Examples of the power of a common vision abound: Steve Jobs achieved unwavering loyalty and commitment from his staff at Apple Computer during the late 1970s and 1980s by articulating a vision of personal computers that would dramatically change the way people lived. The founders of Sony said that in 50 years their brand name would be as well known as any on earth, that it would signify innovation and quality, and that their products would result in "made in Japan" meaning something fine, not something shoddy. Bill Gates envisioned a computer on every desk and in every home. And Jack Welch described a future in which General Electric would be the most profitable, most diversified company on earth, with world-quality leadership in every one of its product lines. In all of these cases, a powerful vision united people to work together toward a common dream.

So the question we wish to address is not whether developing a common vision based on trusting relations matters. It most certainly does. Rather, the questions before us include: How does one build a common vision based on trust and open communication in the face of the fundamental differences between physicians and hospital administrators? And how have efforts to do so fared?

ONE DREAM

Successful collaboration between physicians and hospital administrators depends on their willingness and ability to develop a common dream or vision and work toward it together (Cutis 2001). Only a shared and transcendent purpose can overcome the differences that characterize the groups (Bujak 2003).

It is therefore not surprising that retreats and other mechanisms for creating and disseminating the dream that would unite physicians and administrators have been so popular. The bonding experiences to which these functions lead contribute to the cohesiveness of the groups (Clevenger 2007). In fact, results of a recent national survey (McGowan and MacNulty 2006) completed by 102 hospital CEOs and 61 physician leaders suggest that both groups believe that sponsoring retreats that include senior management and physicians is an effective integration strategy.

It appears to make sense. Spending time together, preferably off-site, generating ideas about who you could become if you moved toward your dream together should promote effective working relationships. After successful retreats, many of you have experienced the euphoria of crafting a dream that seemed to capture everyone's interest and pull everyone together.

But what often happens next? The complaints we hear from hospital administrators and physicians after such events include:

1. *The euphoria doesn't last.* In fact, even the most exciting aspects of the vision often lose their appeal in the harsh light of the real world and its day-to-day challenges.
2. *We can't make it work.* Even if the vision continues to be appealing, it is just too hard to make it work. The details of actually implementing the vision were not addressed at the retreat, and now we have no idea how to do it. In fact, it looks impossible.
3. *We can't sell it to others in our organization.* Even if the vision continues to be appealing, and even if we can see how it could be implemented, too many people in our organization who were not at the retreat do not buy into it. The cynicism from having tried this many times before (unsuccessfully) makes it impossible to bring them along, so the whole effort eventually fades away and becomes one more of those unsuccessful attempts.

Has your organization experienced one or more of these scenarios? Have the failed attempts at dream building left people disillusioned and cynical? To be sure, each failed attempt will likely make it even more difficult to achieve success with subsequent attempts. Sometimes these failures are due to a poorly run retreat or a lackluster vision statement. Often, however, the intended results of even the best-planned retreats are simply unrealistic. Why would conflicting groups with a long history of distrust put aside their differences to follow a dream that is not likely to work anyway?

THE ROLE OF TRUST AND OPEN COMMUNICATION

Trust can be defined as the extent to which one is willing to ascribe good intentions to, and have confidence in, the words and actions of other people (Firth-Cozens 2004). Trust, when it exists, is the social glue that keeps parties together in settings ranging from entrepreneurial start-ups to international joint ventures. Trust makes ventures between differing parties more likely to be resilient and successful (Svejenova 2006). Sadly, almost everyone agrees that physicians and hospital administrators generally do not trust one another, and that this lack of trust is one of the main reasons for their poor relations (Bujak 2003).

In fact, distrust appears to be the norm. In 1999, the Advisory Board surveyed hospital CEOs and physicians to find out what each group felt was most important to itself and to the other (Advisory Board Company 1999). The CEOs said that quality of care was their primary concern, but they thought that physicians were most concerned about their own incomes. Physicians, on the other hand, believed the exact opposite: They cared about quality care, while they thought that CEOs mostly worried about money. Is it any wonder that these two groups do not trust one another?

This trend has worsened over time, with young MDs trusting their hospital partners less than their predecessors did (Anderson 2003). At the same time, hospital administrators do not trust physicians who have entrepreneurial personalities or a strong desire for increased technology, medical equipment, and access to facilities (Holm 2000). So while neither side can survive (much less thrive) without the support of the other, each resents the other (Hekman 2002), each fundamentally distrusts the other, and each views the other as a major source of its problems.

Researchers have documented the development of interpersonal trust in a wide range of industries, including pharmaceuticals, software, financial services, energy, computers, and electronics (Abrams et al. 2003). They have identified interpersonal and organizational "trust builders." Primary among trustworthy interpersonal behaviors was frequent and rich communication. In fact, research long ago indicated that poor communication is the most frequently cited source of interpersonal conflict (Thomas and Schmidt 1976). Specifically within healthcare, Stephen Shortell (1991) emphasized the importance of shared values and open, honest communication for building trust. The prevailing belief, then, seems to be that administrators and physicians can develop trust by applying honest, factual, and timely communication principles—even if there is an underlying competitive reality between them (Howard 2003).

The challenge, of course, is that the same words may mean different things to physicians and to administrators. Speaking to one another and really understanding each other are not the same. Because hospital administrators and physicians view the world through different lenses, they will likely interpret the same observations or the same communication differently (Atchison and Bujak 2001).

Trust is required to accept that another's interpretation of a situation may have some merit. One way to build such trust is to ensure the existence of a shared vision and language (Abrams et al. 2003). But as we noted earlier, creating a shared vision and language depends on trusting relations among the parties. So distrust leads to an unwillingness/inability to forge a common vision and to poor communication patterns, and each of those, in turn, reinforces the distrust, in an ever-strengthening cycle of negative reinforcement, as shown in Figure 3.1.

It is hard to know where to intervene in this self-reinforcing negative cycle, so the most common approach has been to simply admonish and declare that one or more of the elements in the cycle *must* change. For example, "Administrators and physicians *need to* develop mutual trust and respect; or blame *must be* eliminated from the vocabulary" (Cohn, Gill, and Schwartz 2005). Friedman (2003)

Figure 3.1 Where to Intervene?

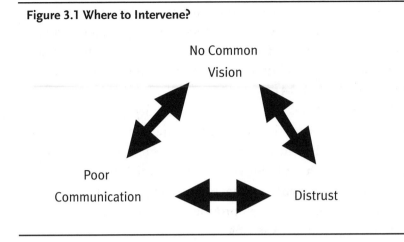

No Common
Vision

Poor
Communication

Distrust

took on all three of the elements of our negative cycle by stating that in order to alleviate the problematic relations, healthcare executives *need to* build trust, take more time and effort to listen to doctors, and make more decisions as a group with improved care for patients as the ultimate vision.

Unfortunately, telling people who distrust one another to trust or to communicate more openly may actually make matters worse. Researchers on prejudice reduction have noted that when people are required to participate in activities designed to change their thinking, they frequently rebel, and the level of prejudice increases (Cotton 2008).

WHY HAVE TRUST-BUILDING/DREAM-WEAVING APPROACHES BEEN SO POPULAR?

Maybe because the United States is such a diverse nation, we want unity above all. We are afraid that our disunity causes our problems. Our overarching social model is the town meeting, where people come together to debate the common good (Gurin et al. 1999). Arthur Schlesinger (1991) summarized the underlying sentiments of this model by stating that when multiculturalism seeks to "discard the idea of a common culture and celebrate, reinforce, and perpetuate separate ethnic and racial communities, then multiculturalism not only betrays history but undermines the theory of America as one people" (13–14).

For much of this country's history, models of intergroup life have called for the muting of differences and the search for integration and unity. It is therefore hardly surprising that the healthcare industry would have followed a similar model in attempting to integrate physician and hospital groups, despite the fact that such an approach may not be appropriate or may actually do more harm than good in this setting.

Unsuccessful Visioning Due to Lack of Trust

As recently as one year ago, it had still seemed possible to get the physicians and administrators at Louis Martin Community Hospital together. Despite their difficulties in dealing with one another, both groups had been angry about the intrusion of payers into their professional lives and had wanted to respond more assertively to these external pressures. At last year's retreat, they had united for the stated intent of controlling the quality of healthcare in their community. Believing that they would now work toward common outcomes that neither could achieve alone, several of their leaders had euphorically assumed that this would help them focus on their similarities and minimize their differences.

Unfortunately, when these leaders returned from the retreat, all did not go as well as they had hoped. The idea of being bound together by this common dream seemed like heresy to many of their colleagues, who wondered cynically behind their backs whether they had been drugged by the mountain air or simply duped by facilitator tricks. Each side saw their leaders as turncoats who had betrayed the interests that they had been sent to serve and had caved in to the other group's demands.

As they prepared for this year's retreat, the administrators and the physicians felt more cautious about their chances of successfully coming together. During the past year, the abstract vision that they had proudly

(Continued on following page)

constructed had crumbled under the misunderstandings that surfaced during implementation. Clearly each group had understood the words to mean something different. While the physicians had expected the dream to lead to an increase in patients and fees, administrators believed it would lower costs, expand referrals, and lead to widespread commitment of physicians to the hospital's well-being.

After much finger-pointing, blaming, and restating how the other side had betrayed their trust, expectations and enthusiasm for this year's retreat were low. In fact, relations between the groups were as bad as they had ever been, and no one believed that one more retreat would make any difference.

WHY HAVE VISIONING APPROACHES FAILED?

Physician–hospital relations are as bad as they have ever been (DeBoer, Iyenger, and Dudhela 2008; O'Connor, Fiol, and Guthrie 2006), despite an acute awareness that the lack of trust between physicians and hospital administrators is a serious issue that must be addressed. More than half of the respondents to a national survey of strategies used to align physicians and hospitals (McGowan and MacNulty 2006) had a formal physician-relations program with professional staff responsible for spending time with active members of the medical staff and their office staffs in an effort to develop trusting relations. A high percentage of the respondents used interviews and print surveys to gain an understanding of physician issues and concerns. But when it came to physicians actually partnering with administrators in running the hospital, there was a large difference of opinion: A majority of the physician leaders responded that it was important for physicians to represent at least 25 percent of the membership of the healthcare system board, while less than half of their CEO counterparts felt the same. This suggests a high awareness of what is needed: trust, respect, open communication, and jointly developed vision and values. It also suggests that we are not getting the results we had hoped for.

Expecting people who fundamentally distrust one another to share a common vision is like expecting historical racial or ethnic enemies to become color blind on command. It does not happen, and attempts to force it to happen inevitably lead to increased intergroup tensions. Why? Because if each group's unique distinctiveness is downplayed to develop a common vision or goal, each is likely to defend its distinctiveness by reacting in a way that restores and highlights the differences. Each group rejects efforts to find commonality and attempts to reestablish its uniqueness that is being ignored.

This pattern will sound familiar to those who have participated in off-site retreats where charismatic and visionary leaders (and consultants) were able to transform difference into commonality by persuasively presenting an overarching vision—only to return to the real world and find that the differences loomed as large as ever. In these cases, the retreat is seldom remembered as more than an exercise in drawing cynicism.

The pattern is not unique to healthcare. A study of math and science students from the same school (Hornsey and Hogg 2000b) showed that emphasizing their school—what they had in common—and downplaying their different disciplines resulted in more intergroup bias, rather than the expected greater sense of commonality. In a similar study of multiple ethnic groups all playing on the same team (Gaertner and Dovidio 2000), downplaying their diversity and emphasizing their common team was associated with greater intergroup bias. The authors of the studies concur that attempts to make members of diverse groups color blind (or blind to disciplinary differences) in order to promote commonality will only lead to counter-attempts to highlight each group's unique differences and to rejection of the perceived imposition of commonality.

Why did visioning approaches work so well in the examples from the beginning of this chapter and not in healthcare? We noted that Steve Jobs's vision of the power of personal computing achieved unwavering loyalty and commitment from his staff, Sony successfully promoted a dream of a powerful brand name, Bill Gates energized his employees with his vision of a computer on every desk and in every home, and Jack Welch described a future for General Electric that engaged his people in their march toward success. Why, then, cannot this same approach be used to pull together physician and administrator groups to work toward a common dream? In the success stories, there were no well-defined lines between essential and interdependent groups who defined themselves as uniquely different and as absolutely not like the "other." As we will delineate in greater detail in the chapters that follow, when the divide between conflicting groups is rooted in fundamentally different group self-perceptions, attempts to promote commonality will most likely be resisted.

CHAPTER SUMMARY

After all of the attempts to structurally integrate hospitals and physicians by placing them in the same bed, and after simultaneous attempts to unite them in trusting collaboration toward a common dream, physician–hospital relations are as strained as they have ever been (DeBoer, Iyenger, and Dudhela 2008). Attempts to emphasize that "we're all in this together" have failed (Budetti et al. 2002). It is time to look in new places for the answers that have seemed so elusive. The next chapter provides an overview of an uncommon perspective for developing hospital–physician collaboration. Although it is based on solid evidence from social psychology and on practical experience, the four-phase approach we describe is not well known within healthcare circles and thus provides a distinct advantage to those who dare to think outside of the box in attempting to develop healthy hospital–physician relations.

SELF-ASSESSMENT EXERCISES

1. Discuss with physicians/administrators how successful your healthcare organization has been in clearly creating, articulating, and building support for a unifying vision.

   How well is this vision known throughout your organization?

   Are decisions consistently made based on this vision and explained/justified as being consistent with this vision?

   To what degree does this vision consistently serve as a unifying theme for physicians and administrators? Is it more appealing to one group than it is to the other?

2. Collect anonymous information regarding your vision from people holding diverse positions throughout your organization (and from those physicians who are not part of the organization).

   To what degree can they clearly articulate your vision?

   To what degree do they understand the implications of your vision for their specific jobs? Does it guide their decision making and behavior on an ongoing basis?

   How proud and inspired are they by the opportunity to participate in the pursuit of this vision?

   Do you notice any significant differences in the responses of physicians and administrators to the above questions? How do these differences affect their ability to work together effectively?

3. Collect anonymous information from people who attended your most recent retreat.

   What do they believe was accomplished? Were these accomplishments meaningfully sustained over time?

Is what was accomplished consistent with your well-articulated vision?

Are the answers regarding what was accomplished similar for physicians and administrators? If not, what differences exist, and what do they imply about any follow-up work that is needed?

4. What values are most important to physicians (administrators) at your organization?

How do physicians' values differ from those of administrators?

What implications do these differences have for the behaviors and outcomes each group prefers?

How do the above answers affect the ability of physicians and administrators to work together effectively?

5. Has your ability to create a common vision for uniting physicians and administrators been affected by poor communication or distrust?

What steps have you taken to enhance trust between physicians and administrators? To what degree have these steps been successful?

What steps have you taken to develop lines of open communication between physicians and administrators? To what degree have these steps been successful?

To the degree that you have been unsuccessful in creating a common vision for unifying physicians and administrators, does that affect the quality of communication and trust at your organization? What actions does your answer suggest should be taken next?

PART II

An Uncommon Approach: Four Phases to Physician–Hospital Collaboration

CHAPTER 4

The Four Phases

What to Do Now?

Collaboration between physicians and administrators at Louis Martin Community Hospital was dead. Conflicts had become a way of life. Mr. Mosher's attempts to form an alliance with the independent physicians had failed even before the partnership was formed. There were simply too many substantive differences and too much negative history for the physicians and hospital administration to reach any agreement.

If that wasn't trouble enough, the recent hospital retreat had been a complete bust. Mr. Mosher had suspected even before the retreat took place that the finger-pointing, blaming, and denigrating behaviors on both sides reflected such a lack of respect for and distrust of the "other" that it was risky at best to bring the warring groups together. But lacking better ideas, he had moved forward with the planned event, a decision he now seriously regretted. The retreat only made the all-out warfare more public. The conflicts were as destructive as ever, and the retreat was seen as one more failed attempt in a whole string of such failures.

When we met Mr. Mosher, he was reeling from a series of failed attempts to stem the conflicts. He had heard rumors that the physicians were initiating a process for removing him from office, and he was seriously considering claiming defeat and simply resigning before they had a chance to do so.

DOES MR. MOSHER'S plight sound familiar? Many factors, including resource allocation decisions, regulatory issues, and pressures from third parties, have contributed to the intergroup conflicts. Physicians and administrators are squeezed in a capital-intensive industry faced with rising consumer expectations, increasing regulations, skyrocketing costs, and declining revenues. Demands abound for better patient outcomes, stronger financial results, and improved staff satisfaction. Of course, significant progress in addressing any of these challenges requires collaboration between physician and administrative groups, so it feels like a hopeless negative cycle from which there is no escape.

The problems plaguing hospital administrators and physicians run deeper and wider than any single individual or group, and they cannot be fixed simply by trying harder at what we have been doing unsuccessfully for decades. Because of the nature of the conflicts between these groups,

- trying to change those "others" who are uncooperative and difficult will only increase their resistance,
- trying to get people to want a change is not enough,
- bringing groups together within an integrated structure typically does not work, and
- getting people fired up about a common vision is frequently a short-term fix at best.

Each of these approaches has been tried over and over with limited success. The fact that you are reading this probably means that you are searching for a new solution to the challenges facing hospital administrators and physicians today.

This chapter provides an overview of the PAR (Physician–Administrator Relations) Process, a novel approach for moving away from the current difficult relations between physicians and administrators that characterize many healthcare settings, and toward healthy and sustainable collaboration.

FOR TRADITIONAL INTEGRATIVE ATTEMPTS TO WORK, YOU NEED SEPARATE TOGETHERNESS

Integrative approaches to collaboration (such as the structural and visioning approaches discussed in chapters 2 and 3) have led to positive results in numerous organizations, including Apple Computer, Sony, Microsoft, and General Electric. But in settings marked by long-standing, entrenched conflicts, reliance on visioning or structural integration is usually futile.

Although it is difficult to argue against bringing the groups together, past attempts have demonstrated that we cannot get there by promoting integrative solutions for groups who are mired in conflicts so deep and divisive that they have actually become part of how the groups define themselves. Earlier in the book we provided detailed evidence that neither the structural nor the visioning approaches for integrating hospitals and administrators have generally proven to be successful. In fact, we demonstrated that promoting contact between the groups and attempting to unite them around a common vision have often torn them further apart.

Integrative vision/goals and structures are threatening because they appear to involve working collaboratively with the enemy. So they are likely to be resisted. Attempts to emphasize that "we're all in this together" when, in fact, each group defines itself, in part, as unlike "them," are like slaps in the face of traditional beliefs; attempts to promote similarity when each group sees itself as fundamentally different is like pretending to be color-blind in the face of racial and ethnic differences. The most likely result of such attempts is counterforce from each of the groups as they try to hold onto their distinctiveness.

Only if physician and administrative groups can maintain their autonomy as separate groups *and* simultaneously unite around a common purpose will traditional approaches result in enduring

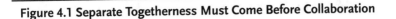

Figure 4.1 Separate Togetherness Must Come Before Collaboration

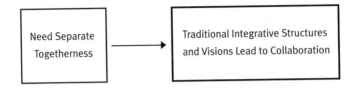

collaboration, as Figure 4.1 illustrates. We call this *separate together-ness*: "togetherness" because the groups collaborate around a common purpose; "separate" because the groups do not sacrifice their unique distinctiveness in the process.

TO ACHIEVE SEPARATE TOGETHERNESS, YOU NEED SEPARATE GROUP SECURITY

Separate togetherness means that group members are committed to the larger unit of which they are a part without giving up the distinctive autonomy of their own group. The groups are like separate ships sailing along parallel paths toward a common destination. But who should captain the healthcare ship—physicians or hospital administrators? Our answer is unambiguous: Each must be the captain of its own ship, and the ships must be aligned on their journey toward a shared destination.

Separate togetherness has led to collaboration in a number of settings. For example, multiple ethnic groups on the same sports team were better able to collaborate for success when they were committed to their own ethnic uniqueness and to the success of the team as a whole (Gaertner and Dovidio 2000). But these ethnic groups were already secure in their own uniqueness before they joined the team. What happens if this is not the case?

Figure 4.2 Separate Group Security Must Come Before Separate Togetherness

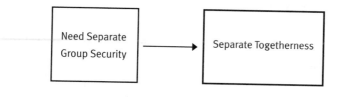

If a group is not secure about its own value and unique contributions to begin with, it will not be able to commit to the vision and goals of a larger unit that includes the former enemy without feeling threatened. Neither physicians nor administrators typically seem focused on the unique value of their peer group. We agree with Bujak (2003), who noted that physicians are not usually united as a group except in their common animosity toward administrators. Fragmented administrative groups, too, find themselves coming together primarily around one of their most pressing concerns, difficult relations with their physicians (Carlson 2009). This means that in most healthcare settings, separate togetherness will not be possible until each group feels secure about its distinctive contributions, as Figure 4.2 shows.

If the physician and administrative groups at your healthcare system are not currently united with their peers and secure in their unique contributions to the system, each group's value and distinctiveness must be promoted before attempting to develop separate togetherness. The purpose of this is to build positive ties among group members who have previously felt little connection to one another except in their common dislike of the "other." It encourages the members of each group to focus on what makes them unique, distinctive, and valuable as a group and to strengthen their ties with each other based on their pride in and satisfaction with being part of such a group.

TO ACHIEVE SEPARATE GROUP SECURITY, THE NEGATIVE CONNECTIONS MUST BE DISENTANGLED

Attempts to strengthen each group's security in its unique value have often led to greater satisfaction for group members. They have also helped to redirect each group's attention from the negative aspects of the "other" to their own positive value. However, at times, such attempts have failed to produce strong positive bonds among group members, and these groups have remained mired in their obsession with the negative "other."

These efforts often fail because it can be threatening to see the distrusted "other" strengthened. Group members may even resist strengthening the bonds among them and promoting their own group's value because it requires letting go of the competitive quirks that have characterized relations among physician specialties or administrative functions. It often seems safer for members of both groups to continue to distrust one another and to individually fend for themselves. Group members may find it difficult to focus on their own group's positive and distinctive contributions if their main connection with others in their group has been their common opposition to the other group. In addition, this negative connection between groups makes the increasing strength and security of the other group seem threatening.

Like fighting dragons that can no longer disengage because the battle has become their identity, physicians and administrators become so engaged in their conflict that it becomes part of how they define themselves. The negative entanglement provides a form of security—if nothing else, the security of the familiar and the certainty that the problems each faces are primarily due to the other. The irony here is that they are often more negatively entangled with the other group than they are positively bonded with others in their own group.

To increase the chances that group members will redirect their attention from the negative "'other" to their own group's positive

Figure 4.3 Negative Connections Must Be Disentangled Before Separate Group Security Can Be Established

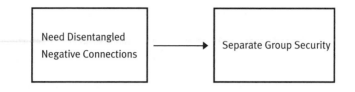

value, it is necessary to reduce the security that comes from the negative entanglements between the groups. Building on evidence ranging from interpersonal conflict management to international diplomacy, we will take you through a process by which the negative ties binding administrator and physician groups together in a locked battle can be broken down, as shown in Figure 4.3, providing an opening for members of each group to cohere around a more positive sense of their unique contributions.

TO DISENTANGLE THE NEGATIVE CONNECTIONS, YOU NEED READINESS TO BEGIN

Some attempts to disentangle the negative connections between groups locked in battle have been highly successful over the long run. Other attempts have broken down before any real progress could be made. The issue is often one of readiness. Are administrators and physicians in your healthcare system ready to let go of the old security blanket called "making the other wrong"?

Readiness to begin (Figure 4.4) means individuals are highly committed to de-escalating the conflict in your organization and demonstrate a steadfast dedication to significantly improving physician–administrator relations. It does not necessarily mean that you *want*

Figure 4.4 Readiness to Begin Must Come Before Disentangling Negative Connections

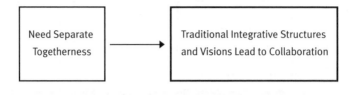

to engage in the processes we are describing. But readiness does mean that you are *willing* to try them, because (1) nothing else has worked, (2) the risks of trying a new path seem lower than the risks of continuing the old ways of relating to each other, (3) you are feeling the negative effects of the ongoing battles between the groups, and (4) you see at least the *possibility* of a new beginning, a new way to relate to one another, and a new way to move toward important healthcare goals.

SHORTCUTS WILL NOT WORK

It is important to emphasize that each of the phases we have described will be successful only if the prior phase has been completed. Only when your groups are ready to take the first steps to change the situation (Phase One) is it possible to engage them in rethinking their relationship; only after the negative connections that have kept the groups enmeshed in their destructive dance have been disentangled (Phase Two) is it possible for each group to feel secure about its unique contributions; and only after each group feels secure in its unique contributions (Phase Three) is it possible for group members to successfully focus on togetherness with the "other" and continued separateness as a distinctive group (Phase Four). Separate togetherness is a foundation for sustained collaboration via traditional integrative approaches, as shown in Figure 4.5. The three dotted arrows

Figure 4.5 Four-Phase PAR Process

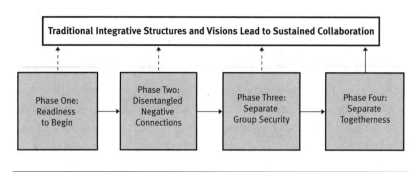

are reminders that the outcomes of the first three phases must continue for collaboration between the groups to be sustained over time; any one of those outcomes alone will not lead to sustained collaboration.

Shortcuts Did Not Work at Louis Martin Community Hospital

At LMCH, the medical staff complained to us that the CEO, Joe Mosher, and his administrative team continued to ignore, and even thwart, patient initiatives and recommendations essential to improving the quality of patient care. This perceived behavior on the part of administration threatened the physicians' collective self-concept (as those having control over medical decisions for their patients). The physicians had responded to that threat by attacking the administrative team's professional identity (as those in control of the organization's future) and refusing to buy into or support its vision for the hospital's future. This behavior had prompted the administrators to withhold further support for physicians' recommendations and had eventually led to the physicians' costly and painful attempts to remove Mr. Mosher. Over time, the original dispute had multiplied exponentially into seemingly unrelated battles, such as fights over allocation of funds.

We were able to temporarily reduce tensions between the physicians and administrators at LMCH through a series of exercises that created readiness to at least consider possibilities beyond all-out warfare. To

(Continued on following page)

capitalize on this initial readiness, we proposed that they initiate three short-term projects that we expected would have recognizable, measurable benefits for both groups. The small group of participants agreed that it would return to the larger group in a few weeks to report its outcomes, ideally demonstrating that the initial group could work together productively, and thus providing a foundation for a follow-up plan. However, the follow-up work to disentangle the negative connections, promote each group's security about its own distinctive value, and create separate togetherness never occurred.

The recognition of the mutual interdependence that the groups gained during the initial projects reduced conflict somewhat in the short run. But agreement on larger initiatives was never reached, and tensions once again began to build. Not wanting to lose the momentum he believed they had achieved, Mr. Mosher had chosen not to engage his people in the intermediate steps we had recommended and had instead reopened conversations about creating a common vision as the basis for reducing the intergroup conflict (moving from readiness to change directly to promoting collaboration). The CEO and the president of the medical staff recognized that the initial readiness had eroded, and that increased cynicism was rapidly taking its place.

At about this time, a survey of several of the competing hospitals in the region ranked LMCH near the bottom in terms of patient satisfaction and the percentage of patients who said they would recommend the hospital to others. Despite the abysmal survey results and the slide back to cynicism and conflict between the groups, Mr. Mosher's goal remained excellence through the eyes of the patients. His goal was laudable. Yet he had not been willing to engage his people in a process that would have given him a chance to achieve it.

WHERE TO BEGIN THE PAR PROCESS?

Chapters 5 through 8 present each of the four phases of the PAR Process in detail. At the end of each chapter, we provide assessment instruments for you to gauge your progress. Some or all of the outcomes of the early phases we describe may already exist in your organization. If this is the case, you may be able to begin your healing with later phases of the process.

Phase One: If there is limited readiness in your healthcare system for people to stop doing the same old thing and to search for a new approach, we recommend that you begin at Phase One, which we describe in Chapter 5. After reading the chapter and completing the self-assessment exercises, you will be able to determine the degree of readiness in your system and whether you need to begin at Phase One.

Phase Two: If your people are truly ready for a change but are still experiencing ongoing battles between the physicians and hospital administrators, we recommend that you begin with Phase Two, which is described in Chapter 6. Although negative entanglement between these two groups is common in many healthcare organizations today, this is not the case in some settings. After reading the chapter and completing the self-assessment exercises, you will be able to determine the need to further disentangle the negative connections between groups at your healthcare system.

Phase Three: If administrators and physicians at your healthcare system do *not* find themselves enmeshed in negative entanglements, it may make sense for you to begin with the third phase, which is described in Chapter 7. Although many physician/administrator groups do not feel a sense of belonging to, or pride and satisfaction in, their group that comes from awareness of their distinctive and unique contributions, you may find that this sense of security is present in your healthcare system. After reading the chapter and completing the self-assessment exercises, you will be able to determine the need to further promote each group's distinctive value in your healthcare system.

Phase Four: If the groups in your health system already feel pride and satisfaction from belonging to a distinctive group of physicians or administrators that adds value to the whole system, you may skip to Phase Four, which is described in Chapter 8. Although it is still uncommon to see people simultaneously committed to the separate autonomy of their own group and its connection with the larger unit, this may be occurring in your organization. After reading the chapter and completing the self-assessment exercises, you will be able to determine the need to further promote each group's separateness and togetherness at your healthcare system.

Table 4.1 summarizes our recommendations about where to begin.

We recommend periodic checks to make sure that the conditions of all of the phases continue to be met. You cannot afford to become complacent; conditions may change before your very eyes and undermine a process you have put in place. For example,

Table 4.1 Where to Begin

Conditions Differ	Where to Intervene?
Physicians and/or administrators in your organization are not ready to do what it takes to change the situation.	Begin at Phase One to develop readiness to begin.
Physicians and administrators are ready to begin, but they are negatively entangled.	Begin at Phase Two to disentangle the negative connections.
Physicians and administrators are not negatively entangled, but they do not feel like they belong to a valued and distinctive group.	Begin at Phase Three to strengthen each group's security about its own distinctive value.
Physicians and administrators feel like they belong to a valued and distinctive separate group, but they do not feel a sense of togetherness with the larger system.	Begin at Phase Four to promote the separate togetherness needed for integrative approaches to lead to sustained collaboration.

assume your assessments indicate that physicians and administrators at your system have successfully gone through Phase One, and you begin the work of Phase Two to disentangle the negative connections between the groups. If none of the efforts to redirect people away from the negative aspects of the "other" are succeeding, things have likely slipped backward, and there may be a need to revisit Phase One before moving on.

Also, beware of assumptions about current conditions in your group or in your system as a whole. In April 2008, the Noblis Center for Health Innovation along with the Eastern Connecticut Health Network presented a program entitled "The Dynamic State of Physician–Hospital Alignment: Practical Strategies to Ensure Your Success" (MacNulty and Reich 2008). They showed that, in 2005, 70 percent of the surveyed presidents/CEOs of hospitals rated relationships between their physicians and administrators as "very positive," whereas only 31 percent of physician leaders rated these relationships that highly. This suggests a large gap between the perceptions of different groups and even among those of members of the same group. Confidence in the results of the assessments in this book requires that you include as many people as possible in the assessment exercises.

WHO SHOULD LEAD THE PAR PROCESS?

Who should lead the PAR Process? When and under what conditions can the leadership of a single group (administrative, physician, or board) guide the process? The answers to these questions vary by the current conditions in your health system and by where you are starting the process. The more deeply entrenched the conflicts in your system are (negatively entangled groups that show little readiness to let go of the battle, for example), the more likely it is that you will require a neutral outsider to help you implement the process. Trust within and between the groups is almost entirely absent under these conditions, so it would be useless at best and self-destructive at worst for the leadership of the physician or administrative groups (or even the board) to attempt to guide people through the process. Table 4.2 summarizes our experience.

Though we suggest the presence of a neutral third party, especially in the early phases, success depends on the active involvement of physicians, administrators, and trustees. For example, in Phase Three,

Table 4.2 Who Should Lead the Process?

Conditions Differ	Who Should Intervene?
Physicians and/or administrators at your organization are not ready to do what it takes to change the situation.	There is no trust. The neutrality of a third party is valuable in Phase One to develop readiness for change. Support from physicians, administrators, and the board is also essential to success.
Physicians and administrators are ready to begin, but they are negatively entangled.	There is no trust. The neutrality of a third party is valuable in Phase Two to help participants disentangle the negative connections. Support from physicians, administrators, and the board is also essential to success.
Physicians and administrators are not negatively entangled, but they do not feel like they belong to a valued and distinctive group.	Leadership from physicians, administrators, and the board is necessary for strengthening each group's security about its unique contributions in Phase Three, with the possible guidance of a neutral third party.
Physicians and administrators feel that they belong to a valued and distinctive separate group, but they are not able at the same time to feel a sense of togetherness with the larger system.	Leadership from physicians, administrators, and the board is necessary for developing separate togetherness in Phase Four, with the possible guidance of a neutral third party.

promoting the distinctive value of the physicians as a group requires the credibility and knowledge of physician leaders, just as promoting the distinctive value of administrators as a group requires these qualities from administrative leaders. And both require the guidance and oversight of the board. This book provides enough information and tools for people in your system to carry out their roles in the PAR Process and to know when outside intervention is needed.

RECOMMENDED ROLLOUT OF THE PAR PROCESS

The PAR Process, like any innovative and initially unfamiliar change, is not likely to diffuse at a uniform rate across your organization. Instead, you should expect a relatively small number of innovators and opinion leaders to consider adopting the process, followed (if you are successful) by an early majority and then the late majority and traditionalists (Rogers 2003). Research on the diffusion of innovations such as the PAR Process suggests that the most powerful channel of influence is not an initial general appeal to everyone in your organization. The majority of your people are more likely to consider adopting the new process if small subsets of people in your organization (innovators and opinion leaders) whom they know and respect have already adopted it. In other words, imitation is the strongest influence channel. This suggests that the most effective way to engage a large number of people in the new process is to first identify and appeal to your innovators and opinion leaders, then reinforce the diffusion to each successive level (to early and late majorities and finally to traditionalists), and to not waste resources on trying to reach a given level before the people at that level are ready to adopt the innovation.

In line with this thinking, the PAR Process begins with the formation of three transition teams—physician, administrative, and board. Each team consists of three to seven opinion leaders (more may be needed if the peer groups are large or highly splintered into subgroups). The roles of these transition teams are to (1) engage with their peers and with members of the other teams in this small-group setting to move through all four phases of the PAR Process and (2) produce observable and measurable results, which provide the basis for larger groups to become engaged in the process while following the transition teams through the phases.

The most important criterion for transition team membership is credibility. If these small groups of opinion leaders are to influence the majority in your organization over time, they must have the credibility to do so. A secondary criterion for transition team membership is a sufficiently open mind to engage in a new way of addressing an old and intractable problem.

The next four chapters describe the consecutive phases of the PAR Process, why each one is important, what it entails, why it is likely to be resisted, how to move through the resistance, and how to produce the intended outcomes of the phase. Each chapter explains how to move innovators and early adopters through the process to achieve the outcomes of that phase, ending with recommendations for how the process may be disseminated to the majority at your organization. The chapters end with assessment tools that allow you to evaluate your progress in achieving the outcomes of the phase and recommended exercises designed to enhance that progress.

CHAPTER SUMMARY

Before engaging in the PAR Process at your organization, it is important to understand the entire process and the purpose of each phase. Chapter 4 provided an overview of the four phases to introduce you to the process. We emphasized that each phase must be completed for the subsequent phase to be successful. We also noted, however, that some of those outcomes may already exist in your organization. We recommend that you read chapters 5 through 8 and complete the self-assessment exercises at the end of each chapter to determine the degree to which your organization has achieved that phase's outcomes. To the extent that it has, you may decide to skip those phases and begin with the next. The assessment exercises at the end of this chapter will give you a sense of how well you understand the overall four-phase process before you consider applying it with innovators and opinion leaders (and later to the majority and traditionalists) at your organization.

SELF-ASSESSMENT EXERCISES

Assessing Your Understanding of the PAR Process

Please respond to each statement by indicating your level of agreement on a scale ranging from Strongly Disagree (1) to Strongly Agree (5).

I understand that attempts to disentangle the conflicts between physicians and administrators are not likely to be successful unless both groups are ready to consider changing their thinking and behavior. _____

I understand that the negative interactions between physicians and administrators must be disentangled before the desired level of security can be developed in each group. _____

I understand that efforts to create separate togetherness are not likely to be successful until both physician and administrator groups are secure in their unique and distinctive contributions. _____

I understand that traditional integrative structures and visions are not likely to be successful until desired levels of separate togetherness have been developed among physicians and administrators. _____

How does your level of understanding look to you when evaluated against these statements? High scores indicate that you have a solid understanding of the process. However, any score lower than four (4) suggests the need to further clarify the process before going forward. What needs to be done to ensure that the PAR Process is clear to you?

_____

_____

CHAPTER 5

Phase One: Develop Readiness to Begin

Hitting the Bottom at Louis Martin Community Hospital

Joe Mosher, the CEO of Louis Martin Community Hospital, was dazed. Dr. Schmidt, president of the medical staff, had just publicly chastised him, saying that he failed to recognize that the practice of medicine had changed dramatically, that he had been in office too long, and that other hospitals were much better at assisting physicians in caring for their patients. Even worse, Mr. Mosher knew that other physicians were sharing similar complaints with the board.

In Mr. Mosher's opinion, the physicians (including Dr. Schmidt) were overpaid, difficult, and ungrateful for the investments he and the board had made in equipment and facilities. He believed that the physicians were driven by their own personal interests and pocketbooks, that they complained too frequently, and that they refused to look at their own failings. The negative attitudes on both sides were affecting morale, turnover, efficiency, referrals, patient care, and the hospital's reputation in the community. Each side believed the other was the source of the problems.

The recent failed attempts to build collaboration between the groups had increased cynicism, adding fuel to a fire that was already burning out of control. A few of the physicians had agreed to engage in several small

(Continued on following page)

(Continued from previous page)

projects with a handful of senior administrators in order to demonstrate that they were ready to find a way out of the destructive patterns. But instead of following the step-wise process we had recommended—from readiness, to disentanglement, to developing each group's security, to separate togetherness—the CEO had opted for a shortcut and had followed the small projects with attempts to get the physicians to buy into a vision for LMCH. This had not only backfired, leaving no possibility of gaining the trust of the physicians, but it had also eroded any trace of optimism that the situation could improve. Physician–hospital relations were at an all-time low.

The administrative and physician leaders at LMCH were locked in righteous conflict. Both sides knew they were right, and neither was able to begin the healing process required to reduce tensions. The two groups found themselves squeezed by rising expectations, increased regulations, skyrocketing costs, and declining revenue, and their inability to work together had brought them to a dead end. They had the same customers, and they were jointly accountable for the health status of their community. But the members of each group were committed to the fact that they were right, that the others were wrong, and that they must continue to defend their positions so that the other group's greed would not destroy healthcare in their community. Any desire to engage productively with the "other" was gone, seemingly for good.

PURPOSE OF THE FIRST PHASE

IT IS HARD to imagine significant progress in clinical quality, patient satisfaction, or economic efficiency at the hospital described above without committed cooperation from the physicians and the administrators. Cold logic alone, however, often fails to produce readiness for change. Intractable righteousness blocks the steadfast dedication needed to improve physician–administrator relations. The purpose of the first phase of the PAR Process is to start moving beyond such costly conflicts by developing readiness to begin the work of de-escalating the conflict in your organization.

WHY IT IS IMPORTANT

Physicians, administrators, and trustees understand the need to control costs to protect the long-term survival of their organizations *and* the need to spend the resources required to improve health and save lives. Understanding of these seemingly paradoxical perspectives, however, does not motivate people to action. Unless people truly desire change, they will seldom take the necessary steps to move beyond their traditional, costly, negatively entangled viewpoints.

Without authentic readiness for change, the idea of common goals and structures will make little sense to physicians and administrators, alignment with the larger unit will be seen as disloyalty, supporting the security of the other group will be viewed as giving aid to the enemy, and efforts to disentangle the negative relations will appear far too risky to command support. Trained to think logically, physicians and administrators often assume that readiness is present and leap past it to engage in strategies that have worked in other settings. However, common strategies such as recognizing the positive contributions of the other group, creating joint ventures, or sharing hospital decision making are likely to be crushed on the rocks of resistance as each group expects the "other" to shift its behaviors to make the strategy work. Progress is unlikely until a burning commitment to change (i.e., readiness) is established so that physicians and administrators are willing to reexamine their own views for the sake of passionately desired progress, rather than continuing to try to impose their will on the "other."

WHAT IT ENTAILS

Readiness to begin a fundamental change such as the PAR Process entails a high level of individual commitment to de-escalating the conflict and dedication to improved physician–administrator relations. Readiness does not require complete trust of the other group, a clearly detailed plan for achieving desired objectives, or seeing the well-being of the other group as important. In fact, the other group is likely to still be perceived as not understanding, greedy, and a threat to your own well-being. Nevertheless, the recognition that "more of the same" will continue to negatively affect financial, clinical, and human outcomes, and the awareness that the organization is losing control of its own destiny to large outside forces, can bring you to a realization that something must change. That recognition, and a willingness to consider how you and your group might behave differently to improve the situation, creates an initial readiness to begin the PAR Process.

WHY IT IS LIKELY TO BE RESISTED

Physician–administrator conflicts waste resources, reduce revenue by diminishing productivity, inhibit the development of new services, hamper recruitment and retention, distract leaders from strategic issues, and drive away patients. It is only reasonable that physicians and administrators would wish to work together effectively to reduce these costs. Why, then, does resistance to change persist in the face of such compelling consequences?

In our work with physicians and administrators we have asked this question on many occasions. Frequent answers include assertions that the "other" fails to recognize or accept the need for change; that other leaders failed to build a compelling case for needed change by providing insufficient communication regarding objectives to be achieved, benefits available, or consequences of failure; or that other leaders have simply failed to manage resistance effectively by beginning and sustaining change on a timely basis. At Louis Martin Community Hospital, for example, prior failed attempts to bring physicians and administrators together had inspired widespread cynicism, blocking any desire to engage in another change process.

Implementing change in healthcare organizations is particularly challenging due to the conflicting interests of diverse stakeholders; the frequent lack of clear, accepted, overarching objectives; and regulatory constraints. But the failure rate for change across all industries is high. More than 65 percent of all major change initiatives fail to realize intended objectives on time and within budget (Cameron 1997; Smith 2002). Healthcare is no exception. Failed quality efforts, reengineering initiatives, mergers/acquisitions, and unsuccessful past efforts to heal physician–administrator relations have left both groups shell-shocked and unenthusiastic about stepping into the next set of proposed transitions. Unresolved grievances, reduced confidence, and a lost sense of control suppress readiness to engage in efforts to improve relations.

Barriers to readiness include the perception that things are not bad enough yet to demand change and the belief that one is too busy handling today's crises to engage in creating a great future. Readiness requires that physicians and administrators be willing to stop blaming members of the other group, stop trying to control the other group, and stop valuing their autonomy and being right more highly than they value patient outcomes and financial stability.

In reality, readiness to invest in improved physician–administrator relations does have short-term costs. For example, physician leaders might have to forgo a portion of short-term earnings to invest the time required to move forward. Administrators have to be ready to invest dollars and time to support the intervention processes. Board members must champion the actions required to cover these costs. Under these conditions, resistance is not surprising.

HOW TO MOVE THROUGH THE RESISTANCE

In the end, mutual readiness for change is unlikely until both groups see either

- a threat to their well-being if they fail to give up their old ways of relating (i.e., shared pain),
- great potential benefits as a result of doing so (i.e., shared gain), or

- decreased danger for themselves as a result of working with the other group (i.e., lowered perceived risk).

Without one of these fundamental inducements, most people are unwilling to move beyond inertia and demonstrate readiness for enduring change.

Picture yourself in a hallway at your hospital. Someone has placed a two-foot-wide board on the floor and placed $10,000 on the end of it, only 15 feet away. Would you walk 15 feet across that two-foot-wide board to pick up $10,000? Most of us would say yes or would rapidly be replaced by someone who is standing behind us, ready to go.

Now, assume the same two-foot-wide board is stretched across an alley between the fiftieth floors of two hotels in New York City. The wind is blowing, and icy rain is falling. Would you walk across that board to pick up the $10,000? Most of us would say no, and when questioned further, would suggest that it seems too risky. What would get people out on that board high in the air? One possibility is a larger reward in the other hotel. For example, if your 18-month-old son had spotted you from the opposite window and was crawling dangerously across, saying "mama, mama," most people tell us they would move rapidly out on the board. Alternatively, if the hotel you are in is on fire, the flames are about to catch on your clothing, the smoke is making breathing next to impossible, and there is no other way out of the room, the board might look like a reasonable possibility. If the risk was reduced by the fire company placing a net only a few floors below the board, many of us would be more willing to venture forth. The same forces (pain, gain, and lower perceived risks) are required to move through the resistance and create readiness for change in your organization (O'Connor and Fiol 1997). We address each one in turn.

Shared Pain

Motivators for reconsidering an entrenched position can include a recent or impending crisis that makes the current course of action too costly to continue. When the building is burning, it is not surprising that people develop a readiness to do something different. Either the pain of the current crisis or leadership sufficiently sophisticated to make people aware of an anticipated crisis can produce this initial readiness to change.

Steps that help to induce readiness through increased pain include the following:

1. Ensure that people are aware of the costs of the continued conflicts. Questions that help increase awareness of the current pain include:

   - What are the specific costs of this ongoing conflict between physicians and administrators?

   - How will your ability to deliver care be affected if no changes occur in physician–administrator relations? The use of resources? The recruitment and retention of staff? The development of new services?

2. Clarify the personal costs for each individual. As long as the costs of the continued conflicts seem to be borne by the "other," the pain will not motivate readiness to change. Questions that make the costs personal include:

   - As a physician, when was the last time an administrator blocked an initiative that was important to you? As an administrator, when was the last time a physician blocked an initiative that was important to you? What happened?

   - What are you regularly not able to accomplish because of conflict with the "other"? What consequences of this are most important to you?

Although pain (or anticipated pain) will encourage people to consider new behaviors, it can also strain tenuous relationships by accelerating an already deteriorating situation. This approach has been used frequently in healthcare (e.g., building a competing facility, revoking privileges), resulting in escalating conflict, rising delivery costs, and bad public relations. Even if physicians and administrators are both in pain, they may not be ready to reconsider their relationship if they still believe other options exist. Instead of putting more pressure on the other people in the situation, it may be more effective to focus on the gains that are possible if the conflicts are resolved.

Shared Gain

Sometimes increased pain actually escalates tensions and promotes seemingly irrational responses. Under these conditions, predicting what the other group will do next is problematic. Focusing on the potential benefits of change may be a more effective way to encourage readiness. At a minimum, it provides a complementary approach that increases the likelihood of achieving the desired results.

Do leaders in your organization tend to focus on the bad things that might happen if physicians and administrators tried to work more collaboratively, or on the possible positive results? As most of us have experienced, we tend to get more of what we focus on. But telling people not to focus on a particular area is ineffective. For example, when you told your young son *not* to hit his little sister, what happened next? Or when you stood over your golf shot begging it *not* to go right and out of bounds, where did it go?

Rather than asking about the source of the problems we are experiencing, which creates a defensive perspective, it may be more effective to focus people on positive possibilities. Steps to induce readiness through a focus on potential gain include the following:

1. Communicate the potential benefits of resolving the ongoing physician–administrator conflicts. Questions that help people become more aware of these include:

- What are the specific benefits of ending this ongoing conflict between physicians and administrators?

- What effect will resolving the conflicts have on your ability to deliver care in the future? On the use of resources? On the recruitment and retention of staff? On the development of new services?

2. Build excitement by clarifying the benefits for each individual personally. As long as the benefits of ending the conflicts are seen as flowing to "others," they will not motivate readiness to change. Questions that personalize the potential benefits include:

- As a physician, what specific things would you be able to do if administrators did not block initiatives that are important to you? As an administrator, what specific things would you be able to do if physicians did not block initiatives that are important to you?

- What would you regularly be able to accomplish if the conflicts were resolved? What would that get you that you really want?

Positive questions such as these lead people to think about building on what is already working rather than defending themselves. This provides them with the experience of helping to create a new and better future.

Lowered Perceived Risk to Reduce Resistance

A final way to encourage readiness in the face of resistance is to reduce the perceived risks of stepping forward to embrace a proposed change. This entails removing the obstacles to moving into readiness for change.

More than four out of five Americans have "only some" or "hardly any" confidence in the people running major corporations (Hurley 2006). Given the history of intractable conflict between physicians and administrators, confidence may be even lower in our healthcare organizations. Not surprisingly, faith, belief, and hope that working with the other group will improve relations are low in many health systems. Under these conditions, the investments required to move forward often do not seem worth the risks involved, resulting in a low level of readiness for change.

To reduce the perceived risks of a change, physicians, administrators, and trustees must first understand what those perceived risks are. They will differ for different people, so the first step is to collect information. Informal meetings, anonymous surveys, or facilitated discussions can reveal the concerns people have about the risks of engaging in a change process. Questions to increase understanding of people's concerns include:

- What worries you most about engaging in a process to improve physician–administrator relations?
- What concerns do you have about speaking openly about the conflicts to a third-party facilitator? To your own peer group? To everyone in the organization, including physicians, administrators, and trustees?
- What would need to be done to reduce the risks of engaging in a process to improve physician–administrator relations?

Creating structural buffers can effectively reduce the perceived risks of changing physician–administrator relations. For example, if either physicians or administrators feel threatened by relationships with the other group and are clinging to negative stereotypes, they are not likely to speak openly in each other's presence or with trustees. To the degree that initial conversations about changing relations can be subdivided, initially buffering the separate groups by having physicians, administrators, and trustees meet separately can be useful.

A similar buffering strategy has been used in international settings to manage multinational teams. For example, an international manager recognized that, for cultural reasons, female Japanese consultants in his organization would not openly participate in large groups or when their male superior was present. Readiness to productively participate increased when the manager broke the team into smaller groups and used a mediator to ensure that the various perspectives were pulled together in the end (Brett, Behfar, and Kern 2006). Similar gains in readiness to participate will likely flow from initially buffering conflicting groups.

Other tools for reducing the barriers to moving forward with the PAR Process address concerns about lack of time and overcommitments. These include

- temporarily removing other duties to allow time for involvement in the PAR Process;
- creating "stop doing" lists to free up the time required for successful participation;
- partially remunerating physicians for their active involvement, if this can be done without lowering their credibility with their peers; and
- facilitating the process with ongoing and timely data collection and feedback, so that people see progress and feel that their time is well spent.

DISSEMINATION OF READINESS BEYOND OPINION LEADERS

Given the psychological (e.g., perceived loss of control) and financial (e.g., investment required) barriers, initial progress toward readiness will most likely come from small groups of visionary leaders who see the potential for long-term payoff for themselves, their patients, and the community. We refer to these people as the innovators and opinion leaders who are on the physician, administrative, and board PAR Process transition teams. Initial conversations need to include agendas appealing to each group's self-interest (e.g., resources, quality of care) to gain support for further conversation.

Observable, measurable progress toward readiness for change by these innovator and opinion leader transition teams will provide the basis for larger groups to become engaged in the process. As we noted in Chapter 4, the majority of your people are more likely to consider engaging in the new process if innovators and opinion leaders whom they know and respect have already done so. This suggests that the most effective way to move a large number of people in your organization toward the readiness for change that the PAR Process prescribes is to direct their attention to the observable readiness of their respected peers on the opinion leader teams.

Progress toward initial readiness on the part of your opinion leaders is not likely to be observable until they actually begin to act on that readiness. The old adage holds here: Actions are more powerful than words. To the extent that early opinion leaders begin to behave differently around the "other," and to the extent that negative stereotyping of the "other" begins to break down, the benefits of the proposed changes will become apparent to the majority, and they will be more likely to come along. In other words, members of the opinion leader transition teams may need to stay one phase ahead of the majority so that their actions and reactions signal to the majority the benefits of following. Before the majority can move toward readiness (Phase One), they may need to see the results of opinion leaders' efforts to disentangle the negative relations between physicians and administrators (Phase Two).

CHAPTER SUMMARY

Readiness for change is required before efforts to de-escalate conflict between physicians and administrators are likely to succeed. Simply understanding the clinical, economic, and human costs associated with intractable conflict is unlikely to move the groups beyond defending traditional viewpoints. A passionate desire for progress (i.e., readiness) must exist before physicians and administrators are willing to reexamine their own views rather than impose them on the other group.

Readiness develops when opinion leaders in each group stop tolerating more of the same and begin considering how they might behave differently to improve the situation. This mutual readiness to change is not likely to occur until physician, administrative, and board leaders recognize that a big threat to their well-being exists if they do not give up their old ways of relating (i.e., shared pain), that great potential benefits will result from doing so (i.e., shared gain), or that there is less danger (i.e., lower perceived risk) associated with working more cooperatively together. This chapter described strategies for creating a state of readiness for changes prescribed by the PAR Process. It provides self-assessment questions for determining your level of readiness, and it suggests exercises for promoting greater readiness in your organization. Only when readiness exists does it make sense to move to the second phase of the PAR Process, disentangling the negative connections, which we turn to in Chapter 6.

SELF-ASSESSMENT EXERCISES

Assessing Your Readiness to Begin

Please respond to each statement by indicating your level of agreement on a scale ranging from Strongly Disagree (1) to Strongly Agree (5).

Past conflicts between physicians and administrators have made our work environment too painful for all involved. _____

We have tried everything we are aware of to deal with the conflicts and are looking for new ideas. _____

There are great possibilities for our healthcare system if physicians and administrators work together more effectively. _____

The physician–administrator conflicts have damaged not only relations between the groups but also patient care and economic outcomes. _____

I am hopeful that there is a better way of resolving physician–administrator conflicts than we have tried in the past. _____

Waiting for members of the other group to change first is likely to perpetuate our problems. _____

The risks of considering new ways of working with the other group are low enough that I am willing to begin doing so. _____

The risks of talking to my peers about new ways of thinking about the other group are low enough that I am willing to begin doing so. _____

How high is your level of readiness to engage in a process of healing the relations between physicians and administrators? High scores indicate that you are ready to begin. However, any response lower than four (4) suggests that this may not be the case. What changes are needed before you can move toward readiness to engage in healing the relations between physicians and administrators?

_____

_____

_____

_____

_____

_____

EXERCISES FOR PROMOTING READINESS

Please set up brief meetings with individuals or small groups of your peers, and carry out the following exercises.

1. Talk with your peers to determine whether they are aware of the clinical, financial, and human costs associated with current conflicts between physicians and administrators. For example:

    Discuss the implications of current physician–administrator relations for the:

    • Care of patients

    • Use of resources

    • Recruitment and retention of physicians, nurses, administrators, and staff

    • Development of new services

    • Identification of a mutually desirable strategic direction

    • Other?

    Do your peers believe that the conflicts between physicians and administrators at your organization have become too painful to continue into the future?

    Do they understand how destructive the conflicts have been, not only to relations between the groups, but also to patient care and economic outcomes?

2. Discuss with your peers what it would be possible to accomplish if physicians and administrators were able to collaborate effectively with one another, and how the work environment would be improved if the conflicts could be resolved.

Do they really believe that there are great possibilities for the delivery of healthcare in your community, if you could just figure out how to improve collaboration between physicians and administrators?

3. Talk with your peers about their major concerns about the risks of collaboration with the "other" group.

How open are they regarding the barriers to more effective relationships? Will they only speak openly about these when the other groups are not present? What happens when the other groups are present?

Do they believe that the risks of considering new ways of working together are low enough that they are willing to begin doing so?

4. In summary, what is your general opinion about the readiness of your peers to engage in the PAR process? What information have you collected that encourages you to believe that their readiness to work to improve relations is high? What issues must still be addressed before they are ready to move forward?

_____

_____

_____

_____

_____

_____

_____

_____

CHAPTER 6

Phase Two: Disentangle the Negative Connections

Pain-Induced Readiness to Begin at Louis Martin Community Hospital

The conflicts between the president of the medical staff and the hospital CEO at LMCH were now legendary. The incident that had set off the most recent round of clashes was Dr. Schmidt's highly public accusation that Mr. Mosher, the CEO, was out of touch with the needs of physicians in the twenty-first century. Now other physicians were siding with Dr. Schmidt, and Mr. Mosher was preparing for all-out warfare.

Clashes between physicians and administrators had a long history, so this was nothing new, except that the conflicts were now public and were affecting almost every aspect of healthcare delivery at LMCH. Leaders on both sides continued to escalate their differences by publicly pointing out how the other needed to change for the good of the hospital. Each made the other out to be wrong about almost everything, each was stuck in its position, and each contributed relentlessly to the failure of the organization.

When Dr. Schmidt and several of his colleagues began talking about building an ambulatory surgery center that would compete with LMCH, Mr. Mosher knew that things had come to a head. The situation had become so painful for everyone involved that radical change was needed. We were asked to come back and reimplement the change process that had been cut short. The pain was severe enough that the majority of the medical staff

---

(Continued on following page)

(Continued from previous page)

and the administrative personnel were desperate for a new solution. Most of them believed that LMCH could do great things if physicians and administrators could figure out how to quit opposing one another.

THE SITUATION AT LMCH was sufficiently painful that most agreed that drastic change was needed if the parties were going to continue to work together. Readiness to engage in the needed change was increasing, because no other viable options seemed available, and because most people believed in the positive possibilities for the physicians and the hospital if they could relate more effectively to one another. Readiness, however, is only an opening for the changes that must occur for physicians and administrators to extricate themselves from their destructive dynamic; it does not mean that the negative entanglements have dissipated. Despite their readiness, the physicians and administrators at LMCH continued to hold the "other" responsible (if not publicly, then certainly in private) for all that went wrong at the hospital. Each held strong negative stereotypes of the other that were activated every time a problem arose: "There they go again; that is what they always do." On the one hand, these stereotypes helped them cope with the stressful conditions of the conflict; on the other hand, they perpetuated the conflict by promoting the zero-sum view that if "we" are right, "they" must be wrong.

PURPOSE OF THE SECOND PHASE

Entangled negative connections can breed a culture of resignation that depletes the energy needed for making changes and holding people accountable. Projects that should take six months to implement drag on for two years, and dysfunctional people become titans, dominating their surroundings for their own advantage because the energy required to rein them in is missing. These conditions can slowly come to be accepted as ordinary, just as they do in a dysfunctional family in which Pop hits Mom and Mom sees the violence as normal and fails to take action to stop it. Merely disentangling these negative connections will not create accountability. Without disentangling them, however, the creation of new levels of accountability for improved outcomes is unlikely.

The purpose of the second phase is to disentangle the negative connections between the conflicting groups by breaking down the stereotypes that have locked them into zero-sum perspectives. It may seem that the conflicting parties are disconnected from one another, but in reality they are tightly connected in ways that are difficult to disentangle. This is illustrated by a personal communiqué sent by Soviet Premier Nikita Khrushchev to President John F. Kennedy at the height of the Cuban Missile Crisis. Khrushchev cautioned Kennedy that the escalating conflict between their countries could be likened to a rope with a knot in the middle of it. "The harder you and I pull, the tighter this knot [of war] will become," he suggested. "And a time may come when this knot is tied so tight that the person who tied it is no longer capable of untying it" (Kennedy 1969, 81). It is futile to attempt to untie the knot while the rope is being pulled from each side. At that point, severing the connection (letting go of the rope and separating instead of attempting to untie the knot) may be necessary.

The results of most recent ethnic civil wars also point to the difficulty of "untying the knot." Of 27 ethnic civil wars that have occurred between 1944 and the mid-1990s, only 8 have ended with a peaceful reconciliation among the parties involved (in 12 cases, one ethnic group won; five territories were partitioned; and two were militarily occupied by a separate country) (Kaufman 1996).

Ultimately, the conflicting groups in healthcare cannot permanently defeat each other, nor can they remain separate, given their interdependence. But when the negative connections, such as those at LMCH, choke off any possibility of discovering common ground, separation (letting go of the rope) must occur before the groups can learn to interact in more effective ways. Isn't it time to stop pulling on the knot?

WHY IT IS IMPORTANT

As long as physicians at your organization see administrators as the source of the problems and vice versa, it is not likely that either group has any real sense of its own unique value. In other words, focusing on the negative "other" keeps you from focusing on your own positive value. Your value comes to be defined in opposition to the "other" rather than reflecting the accomplishments of your own group. Negative stereotypes keep both groups from feeling a positive sense of their own group's uniqueness.

The importance of breaking down the negative stereotypes that keep conflicting groups locked in intractable battles and introducing the complexity of a situation to participants who have long lived in an overly simplified, polarized world has been demonstrated in numerous settings, including international diplomacy (Kelman 1997) and family therapy (Public Conversations Project, n.d.). For example, Herbert Kelman (now retired professor of social ethics at Harvard University) devoted his career to de-escalating the conflicts between Arabs and Israelis. His disentangling efforts entailed nonofficial workshops with third-party mediators that had a dual purpose. One was to get participants to develop a more differentiated view of their opponents. For physicians and administrators, this would mean recognizing that all physicians are not the same, nor are all administrators. The second purpose was to ensure that the new understandings developed in the workshops fed back into each community (Kelman 1997). Participants came to his workshops firmly believing that the fulfillment of the other's national identity meant the destruction of their own and vice versa—certainly an extreme illustration of the power of negative stereotypes to keep people stuck in their positions. Kelman's work was not a substitute for official diplomacy efforts, and disentangling the negative connections does not mean that conflicts have been resolved, as history has demonstrated. Nevertheless, Kelman's disentangling work was a central part of diplomatic processes in the Middle East, paving the way for more formal negotiations (Fisher 1997). Similarly, disentangling the negative connections is not the final solution to the conflicts in your organization, but it does pave the way for engaging your people in the subsequent phases of the PAR Process, eventually leading to healing and collaboration between the groups.

WHAT IT ENTAILS

Disentangling the negatively entwined groups entails creating awareness that one group does not have to lose for the other to win. It is about directing people's focus away from what "they" are not doing or what "they" are doing wrong. Groups that have long been engaged in hostility and conflict often take on a "get them before they get us" attitude, and it becomes a big part of how they see themselves and their roles. Disentangling requires a willingness to take suspicious eyes off the "other," to let go of old stereotypes, and to accept that there are additional ways of viewing the "other." Disentangled groups are able to see things from a new perspective and to see others as multidimensional, which allows them to consider the possibility that everything "they" do does not have to be bad in order for "us" to be good.

We recommend a three-step process for disentangling. The first step encourages the understanding that the situation may not be zero-sum—that is, it may not be necessary for one group to lose for the other to win. The second step teaches people to engage in constructive dialogue, which entails listening to understand the beliefs and concerns of the "other" and communicating uncertainties and deeply held beliefs. The third step involves collaboration in a limited set of "small wins," projects that demonstrate the positive outcomes that can result from working together.

Finding Common Ground

The first step in the untangling process involves finding similarities that the groups may share despite their many differences. The purpose of this step is to differentiate the groups' views of each other sufficiently that they see that *all* their aspirations and desires are not at cross-purposes. The purpose of this step is not to build a common dream, but simply for the groups to realize that their worldviews are not entirely black and white.

This step entails initially separating the teams and asking members of each transition team (i.e., physicians, administrators, trustees) to identify the five to ten issues that are most important to them professionally. These may include error reduction, cost containment, the hospital's reputation, or other professional issues. After each group has separately identified a list of issues, the groups are combined and the lists are shared. People are encouraged to identify any common items among the lists.

If the lists appear to not overlap, one option is to identify causal links that participants may not have considered. For example, the positive relationship between error reduction and the reputation of the hospital or health system can be emphasized. The point of this exercise is for participants to realize that a zero-sum perspective of each other is inaccurate, and that some consistency exists among their viewpoints.

Constructive Dialogue

Once people recognize that some areas of overlap exist among the groups, and that win-win solutions might be possible, you can build on that recognition by engaging people in a new way of relating to one another. We have found that some methods family therapists use for teaching the art of constructive dialogue can be applied to the public arena. For example, in 1989 the Family Institute of Cambridge initiated the Public Conversations Project (PCP) to explore the possibility that their ways of working with intense interpersonal conflict could be adapted for use in the public arena. The project's emphasis is not on resolving specific disputes but rather on improving the way people with strong differences relate to each other. In their words, it is about *transformation* rather than *resolution*. Their experience has been promising, often transforming the relations among bitter opponents (e.g., pro-life and pro-choice groups) from polarized diatribes to sensitive dialogues about divisive issues. In addition to its work on abortion issues, the PCP has been involved in conflicts involving sexual orientation and faith traditions, Arab–Jewish and interfaith relations, environmental concerns, social class, population and women's health, and the red/blue divide.

We can draw a number of lessons from their experience. Table 6.1 lists some of the ways that their dialogues differ from destructive debates that have tended to characterize the groups with whom they have worked.

Table 6.1 Destructive Debate Versus Constructive Dialogue

Destructive Debate	Constructive Dialogue
Pre-meeting preparation is minimal.	Pre-meeting contacts and preparation of participants are essential elements of the process.
Participants tend to be leaders known for propounding a carefully crafted position.	Those chosen to participate are not necessarily outspoken leaders (in fact, they should usually not be, because such people tend to be the most polarized in their thinking). They speak as individuals whose experiences differ in some way from others on their side (e.g., administrators who have had both good and bad experiences with physicians).
The atmosphere is threatening; attacks are expected.	Facilitators propose, get agreement on, and enforce clear ground rules to promote respectful exchange.
Participants speak as representatives of groups.	Participants speak as individuals, from their own unique experiences.
Differences within "sides" are denied or minimized.	Differences among participants on the same side are revealed.

(Continued on following page)

(Continued from previous page)

Destructive Debate	Constructive Dialogue
Participants express unwavering certainty and commitment to their point of view.	Participants express uncertainties, as well as deeply held beliefs.
Participants listen in order to refute the other side's data. Statements are predictable with little new data.	Participants listen in order to understand the beliefs and concerns of the other. New information surfaces.
Success requires simple impassioned statements.	Success requires exploration of the complexities of the issues being discussed.

Here are some guidelines for how such a process might unfold at your organization.

1. Pre-meeting preparation includes communication about issues related to the process: What do you hope to achieve through the dialogue? Should the dialogue be a single session, a series of sessions, a two-hour session, a two-day retreat? What should the group size and composition be? Who will facilitate and convene?

2. Commonly used ground rules include:

   • We will speak for ourselves and allow others to speak for themselves, with no pressure to represent or explain a whole group.

   • We will not criticize the views of others or try to persuade them.

   • We will listen with resilience, "hanging in" when something is hard to hear.

   • We will ask questions to check out assumptions we are making.

- We will share airtime, not interrupt, and "pass" if we are not ready or willing to respond to a question.

- When discussing our experience in the dialogue with people who were not present, we will attach no names or other identifying information to particular comments.

3. In divisive, destructive debates, people often state well-entrenched positions (over and over and over) and give arguments to support those positions. In order to stimulate a constructive dialogue (designed for learning rather than winning), use questions that invite people to communicate something other than the "same old, same old." The "new" is fostered by questions that ask you to:

- speak personally, rather than as representatives of a group;

- share stories about the way that your life experiences may have shaped your views;

- shift from expressing positions to expressing hopes, fears, values, and assumptions;

- speak about uncertainties, complexities, and gray areas in your views in addition to what you know for sure;

- explore buzzwords or emotionally charged terms that hold different meanings for different people;

- reflect on your assumptions; and

- expand the range of experiences and information that you pay attention to and share with others.

Such dialogues can promote healing when people are struggling with a deeply entrenched controversy. They counter our tendencies to gravitate to people who share our views and to make public announcements that present the most offensive representation of the other side. As we become selectively informed, we become selectively ignorant and less able to appreciate the extent of our ignorance. Constructive dialogues begin to bridge costly divides born out of such ignorance, leading to the possibility of seeing that the two groups may share some common ground.

Small Wins

Finally, how can small groups of physician and administrative leaders establish the level of confidence required to let go of the tightly knotted rope? Projects that result in small wins for both groups offer one proven route to success. For example, in one organization we worked with, the hospital medical staff was united in complaining that administrators ignored or thwarted its recommendations that were essential to quality care, felt invalidated by their loss of control, and retaliated by attacking the CEO's vision and demanding his removal. Administrators countered by withholding support from further physician recommendations and launching a community public relations campaign that criticized the physicians. Despite the ongoing damage, both groups continued to pursue their own interests separately as the annual physician, administrator, and board retreat approached. As a facilitator for the retreat, what would you do to untangle the negative relationships?

Short-term, confidence-building, small-win projects provide one means of breaking down the stereotypes that keep intractable conflicts alive (O'Connor and Bujak 2001). Characteristics of these projects include

- being doable,
- providing desired benefits for physicians and administrators,
- providing opportunities for early wins, and
- thoroughly clarifying expectations in advance for physicians, administrators, and trustees by

- specifying how success will be measured,

- clearly defining physician and administrator owner-ship and accountability, and

- clarifying how and when results will be reported.

One such project jointly undertaken by one physician and one administrative leader at Louis Martin Community Hospital required altering established supervisory practices to improve clinical outcomes and financial results on a particular hospital floor. The physician had pushed the project idea for months, and it had become a reality. He and his administrative partner formed a clear set of agreements about clinical and financial measures of success, when the successes would be assessed, and how the results would be communicated to their colleagues. Naturally, board interest in and commitment to the project were important to its success.

The small wins project at LMCH provided positive results for physicians and administrators, creating credibility and providing a new view of the "other." We suggest attempting several such projects simultaneously, since a single project may not produce the positive outcomes that help break down the negative stereotypes these groups hold of one another. A series of small wins can provide a foundation for de-stereotyping and for more differentiated views of the former "enemy."

Collaboration with the "other," even on small projects, can seem risky if the entire history of the relationship has been pulling tightly on your side of the knotted rope to keep the "other" from winning. Negotiation research has suggested "graduated reciprocation" (Osgood 1962) for inducing each side to let go of the knotted rope when untying it has become impossible. A sequence of carefully calibrated and clear signals selected to reduce tension can break down mutual antipathy and distrust. This approach has attracted attention because it seemed to offer a mechanism for reducing distrust and suspicion between the nuclear superpowers in the 1960s. Several practical recommendations have come from this work:

- Selected initiatives should demonstrate your commitment to reducing tension between the groups.
- Plans should be announced ahead of time, and the initiative should be carried out as announced.
- Initiatives should be irrevocable and noncontingent so they are not seen as attempts to gain a quid pro quo.
- Initiatives should be continued for a period of time, giving the other party time to rethink its position.
- Initiatives should be noticeable and unexpected to provoke attention and thought.

WHY IT IS LIKELY TO BE RESISTED

Disentangling groups that are mired in the sorts of conflicts physicians and administrators often experience is challenging for three reasons. First, the entanglement is not between individual physicians and individual members of an administrative staff (though individual differences may exist). Individual conflicts can be dealt with using standard conflict-resolution tactics. In conflicts between groups, a widespread collective grip pulls the rope, creating an ever-tighter knot. Negative group-level stereotypes may exist even in the face of positive interpersonal relationships. All physicians may be seen as the enemy in the cost-cutting battles of hospital administrators, despite positive relationships between certain physicians and certain administrators. Da Ponte makes this point clearly in Mozart's *Cosi Fan Tutte*. Don Alfonso exclaims: *"E'la fede nelle femmine come l'Araba Fenice, che vi sia ciascun lo dice, dove sia nessun lo sa."* And the lovers respectively respond: *"La Fenice e Dorabella"* and *"La Fenice e Fiordiligi."* In complete and mutual contradiction, they boldly accuse all women of being unfaithful, except their own fiancées! Individual cases that do not fit with ingrained stereotypes are easily dismissed as exceptions to the rule.

Second, these conflicts are rooted in each side's collective and historical narratives. History will not allow people to loosen their grip on biased perceptions about the way things are. The memories of the atrocities of the fourteenth-century Turkish conquest of Kosovo were still playing themselves out 600 years later in the conflict between Albanians and Serbs (Troebst 1998). And the collective memories of the 1948 Arab-Israeli War, known to the Israelis as the "War of Independence" and to the Palestinians as the "Catastrophe," have fueled continuing battles over the years (Tamari 2002). What are the collective memories of physicians and administrators at your hospital, and how do they replay themselves in self-sustaining ways, over and over again?

Third, these conflicts are rooted in deep-seated beliefs each side holds about itself (we are right; we know what needs to be done) and about the adversary (they are wrong; they do not understand what has to happen). Just as in tribal wars that last for generations, such collective beliefs are perceived as unquestioned truths, which means, by definition, that they are highly resistant to change.

It is not surprising, therefore, that parties engaged in such conflict would resist being stripped of the security that the constant opposition provides. How can opposition provide security? When parties are locked in a zero-sum battle in which one party's gain depends on the other party's loss, the only way to be secure about being right is to keep that battle alive. Kelman (1983) published a report on two lengthy interviews he held with Yasser Arafat, then chair of the Palestine Liberation Organization. The article and its author were immediately attacked by Israeli critics, who viewed it as cavorting with the enemy. A similar pattern plays itself out in many healthcare organizations today. Members of either group risk being viewed as traitors by their peers if they openly try to understand the views of the "other" or work with them on projects designed to produce benefits for all involved.

If nothing else, the negative entanglement provides the security of the familiar, and of knowing that someone else is to blame for the problems you face. The unquestioned certainty that the "other" is responsible for your problems supports the view that the situation is beyond your control, allowing you to see yourself as good and the "other" as bad. You thus preserve a positive self-image and the comforting view that there is nothing you need to change. It is hard to let go of the security and control that the familiar negative entanglement provides. When distrust is severe, why would you think you could afford to quit focusing on everything that the "other" does wrong?

HOW TO MOVE THROUGH THE RESISTANCE

If resistance to disentangling the negative connections is high at your organization, it may not be possible to engage people in the three steps we outlined earlier for finding common ground, learning to interact via constructive dialogue, and identifying joint initiatives for small wins. We have found the approaches that follow useful for moving people through the resistance.

Transfer of Learning

Rather than asking people to step into the others' shoes, which may simply increase resistance, have people study a conflict that is not their own. For example, 68 twelfth-grade Israeli-Jewish students studied the Northern Ireland conflict for a few weeks (Lustig 2002). Though the analogy to their own conflicts was likely apparent, it was not made explicit. At the end of the study, the students were asked to write an essay about their own conflict from the Palestinian point of view. Those students who participated in the study of the remote conflict were able to write well-balanced and impartial essays using the first person, but only a handful of nonparticipants wrote anything at all. Those who did, wrote third-person essays filled with negative expressions. This process for gaining perspective is referred to as *transfer of learning*, and the concept behind it is that something learned in an emotionally neutral context can be transferred to a more emotionally loaded context.

At your organization, this might entail having the three transition teams (administrators, physicians, and trustees) meet separately to discuss conflicts that are affecting organizations other than your own (e.g., symphony musicians and their board, labor unions and management). Similar intractable disputes characterize those relationships, and lessons may be transferred to increase understanding of the conflicts closer to home. After identifying the entangled stereotyping and discussing recommendations for de-stereotyping in the other organization, physicians, administrators, and trustees can meet to discuss shifting the stereotyping and conflicts at your own organization. An example of such an exercise that we have used successfully to disentangle negative connections between physicians and administrators (based on the conflicts between management and unions at United Airlines) is presented in an exercise at the end of this chapter.

De-stereotyping

The PCP, described earlier in this chapter, also provides lessons for working through potential resistance. Like Kelman's work in the international arena, the PCP approach disrupts stereotyping and introduces to participants the complexity of the situation. The therapists describe an effective de-stereotyping exercise in which, rather than asking people to characterize the "other," they ask members of each group to list the negative stereotypes they believe others hold about them. This way, stereotypes are aired without one side derogating the other. After the therapists collect the stereotypes, they ask the individuals or groups who drew up the lists to indicate which stereotypes they consider most inaccurate, inaccurate but understandable, and most painfully accurate. This process raises awareness of the damage the stereotyping has caused for everyone involved. The exercises at the end of this chapter provide additional guidance for moving people through the de-stereotyping process at your organization.

DISSEMINATION OF DISENTANGLEMENT
BEYOND OPINION LEADERS

Initial progress toward disentangling the negative connections between hospital administrators and physicians is likely to flow from the small groups of innovators and opinion leaders on physician, administrator, and board PAR Process transition teams. As the majority in the organization witness constructive dialogue taking the place of (often public) destructive debates, and as they see the positive results of the small wins projects, their readiness to engage in the process themselves will likely increase.

The deep distrust that characterizes the relationships between the groups is initially difficult to invalidate. In fact, it can be self-fulfilling, generating a reality that is consistent with itself. For example, at Louis Martin Community Hospital, Mr. Mosher was initially certain that the physicians would not continue to carry out the small wins projects we had recommended. Based on this certainty, he at first did not follow through with the process. Of course, this then allowed the physicians to complain that Mr. Mosher was, as usual, failing to fulfill his promises. The mutual distrust generated realities that fit well with preconceived stereotypical views. It then became completely rational to behave accordingly, even for those without direct experience. At such a point, a third party may be needed to set up or restart experiments to determine whether the distrust is founded (Gambetta 1988). In addition, board commitment and follow-up to ensure that agreements are kept are important to continued success.

Third parties can play a significant role in letting go of deeply ingrained negative relations and in publicly disseminating the outcomes. Mediators can inject new norms, routines, and procedures that can help people rethink the way they interrelate. In the small wins experiment at LMCH, little progress was made until an outside intervention moved them—at least temporarily—toward recognizing the consequences of their behavior and the possibility of positive expectations for a limited set of low-risk projects. Without the baggage (i.e., distrust, animosity) that comes with a history of intractable conflict, an outsider is often in a better position to ask questions and initiate activities that point physicians and administrators toward recognition of the negative stereotyping on both sides.

Third parties may also pick up on nuances of subtle changes in the relationship that might be cause for celebration. One of the tenets of disentangling is a determined effort to prevent reenactment of the habitual, unproductive ways of relating and communicating and to foster the new. Not surprisingly, the new is often elusive and can take forms that are hard to describe—a thought barely emerging, a distinction on its way to being drawn, or an opinion so out of keeping with convention that it can easily be missed. Third-party facilitators are typically better able to pick up on the new opinion or the new distinction and to help groups to build on them.

CHAPTER SUMMARY

Although conflicting groups may appear to be disconnected from one another, they are often tightly negatively connected in ways that are difficult to disentangle. If you have historically defined yourself by your opposition to the other, you are in fact negatively connected to that other in ways that keep you locked in zero-sum views of the other.

This chapter described how you can begin to disentangle the negative connections by taking a more differentiated view of the other. Constructive dialogue and positive results from small wins projects can move your organization from destructive stereotyping to healthy debate. You are then poised to begin Phase Three of the PAR Process, strengthening separate group security, which we turn to in Chapter 7.

SELF-ASSESSMENT EXERCISES

Assessing Your Level of Disentanglement

Please respond to each statement in Sections 1 and 2 by indicating your level of agreement on a scale ranging from Strongly Agree (1) to Strongly Disagree (5). Average the scores for each section separately. Depending on who is completing the assessment, Section 1 will provide information about how physicians actually view administrators *or* how administrators and trustees believe physicians view administrators. Similarly, Section 2 will provide information about how administrators actually view physicians *or* how physicians and trustees believe administrators view physicians.

Section 1: Physicians

Physicians believe that administrators are stuck in their current viewpoints regarding physicians.   _____

Physicians believe that controlling administrators is necessary to their own success.   _____

Physicians have difficulty getting the information they need to be effective from administrators.   _____

Physicians do not take responsibility for their own contributions to the organization's problems.   _____

Physicians feel angry about the behavior of administrators at the organization.   _____

Physicians do not attempt to really understand why administrators might feel peeved or disgruntled.   _____

Average score for Section 1   _____

Section 2: Administrators

Administrators believe physicians are stuck in their
current viewpoints regarding administrators.   _____

Administrators believe that controlling physicians is
necessary to their own success.   _____

Administrators have difficulty getting the information
they need from physicians to be effective.   _____

Administrators do not take responsibility for their
own contributions to the organization's problems.   _____

Administrators feel angry about the behavior of
physicians at the organization.   _____

Administrators do not attempt to really understand
why physicians might feel peeved or disgruntled.   _____

Average score for Section 2   _____

If you are a physician, the average score of Section 1 reveals how
you view administrators; if you are an administrator or a board
member, the average score in Section 1 reveals your opinions about
how physicians view administrators.

If you are an administrator, the average score of Section 2 reveals
how you view physicians; if you are a physician or a board member, the average score in Section 2 reveals your opinions about how
administrators view physicians.

How does your organization look to you when evaluated against
these statements? High scores indicate that your organization may
have successfully done the work required to disentangle the
entrenched conflict between physicians and administrators. Average
scores lower than four (4) suggest that these relationships need more
healing. What changes are needed to further disentangle the negative interactions between physicians and administrators?

EXERCISES FOR PROMOTING DISENTANGLEMENT

If people are highly resistant to disentangling the negative connections, please begin with the following two exercises:

1. Collect information on intractable conflict between groups in another setting (e.g., labor unions and management).

   Discuss the characteristics of this other conflict, noting especially each group's negative stereotypes of the "other."

   As an independent outside observer of this other conflict, how would you recommend that these groups move beyond their zero-sum view of each other?

   Discuss how your recommendations for the labor–management dispute might be relevant to your own conflict.

   An example of such an exercise (based on the conflicts between management and unions at United Airlines presented in the box) follows.

Management–Union Strife at United Airlines (1980s–2008)

In 1985, United Airlines' pilots went on strike to protest the strategies their CEO was pursuing. Since then, employees (especially members of the ALPA and IAM unions) have been openly critical of the management team. Original disputes between pilots and the management team were about job security and wages. Over time, the conflicts have spread to other areas, including mergers and acquisitions, the dropping of Pacific routes, issues of employee ownership, and issues associated with the company's bout with bankruptcy. Employee–management conflicts have expanded over time to include an increasing number of unions (e.g., flight attendants). The conflicts have continued over the years, becoming especially fierce after 2002, with United's filing for and subsequent emergence from bankruptcy.

(Continued on following page)

(Continued from previous page)

United's management team has tended to view pilots and other employees as having little to no understanding of finance and corporate strategy. Many of the employees, by contrast, have viewed management as too self-interested and uncaring. They feel that management has done little to protect them, does not understand the airline culture, and has been too bottom-line driven. These views have been made very public, leading to open antagonism between the groups.

Despite the damage poor employee–management relations have done to the airline, management teams and labor unions have often continued to pursue their own interests separately with one's gains seen as the others' losses. For example, pilots and some other employees believed that the management team's ventures into mergers and acquisitions came at a cost to their seniority system and their jobs. The management team, by contrast, blamed employees for failures in these endeavors.

Both groups have disparaged the other side, openly and publicly. For example, one article stated, "Management says United is dragged down by the most expensive labor contracts in the business. The unions maintain that management has made several horrendous business moves, especially an ill-fated attempt to buy U.S. Airways that was blocked by the Justice Department last year. Now, they say, United is making another by threatening a bankruptcy filing, a move that would probably wipe out the value of UAL stock" (Wong 2002).

In summary, the implications of the above are that the management team has often defined itself as unlike the pilots and other employees who are viewed as caring about their own interests rather than about the company's future profitability, and that pilots and other employees have not been able to relate to managers who they believe do not understand the nature of the industry or the work of the employees.

a. List the key characteristics of the management–union conflict described in the box, noting especially the negative stereotypes that each group uses regarding the "other."

_____

_____

_____

b. As an outside observer of this conflict, how would you recommend that these groups begin to move beyond their
   zero-sum views of one another?

_____

_____

_____

_____

c. How might your recommendations for the United Airlines
   labor–management dispute be relevant to the stereotyping
   and conflicts between physicians and administrators at your
   organization?

_____

_____

_____

_____

d. Please share and discuss your recommendations with peers
   in your transition team. What recommendations were most
   common? How can they be applied to shifting the stereotyping and conflicts at your organization?

_____

_____

_____

_____

e. Go through the same exercise with other members of your peer group.

2. Ask physicians and administrators to meet separately and complete the following tasks: List the negative stereotypes you believe the other group holds about you. Specifically, as physicians, how do you believe administrators view your group as contributing to the problems in your healthcare system? As administrators, how do you believe physicians view your group as contributing to the problems in your healthcare system? (Note that this is different from sharing the stereotype your group really holds of the other group, which is best put off until work in Phase Three of the PAR Process has enhanced security within each of the groups.)

Clarify in your separate groups what you believe has led the other group to hold these stereotypes about your group. Which of these stereotypes do you believe to be most inaccurate, inaccurate but understandable, and most painfully accurate? Why?

List the ways your beliefs about how the other group views you have influenced your behaviors and blocked efforts to collaborate.

With ground rules and a facilitator to ensure an environment of learning (versus blaming), meet with members of the other group and share your list of stereotypes you believe they hold about you and the way these beliefs have influenced your behaviors and efforts to collaborate. Give them the opportunity to fully understand your list (rather than disagree over it or add to it). Encourage them to repeat back their understanding of what you have communicated and gather new information until you acknowledge that they do fully understand what you have communicated. Note any changes that may occur in your lists as they are repeated back to you.

Share the information exchanged in the above exercise with board members so that the assumed stereotypes and their behavioral implications are clear to everyone involved without blaming or finger-pointing.

As resistance lessens and people become more aware of the damage their negative stereotypes have caused, they are likely to be more ready to engage in the following three exercises for further disentanglement.

3. Ask physicians, administrators, and board members to meet separately and list the five to ten issues that are most important to them professionally. Include in the list the goals your group believes to be most important for your healthcare system to accomplish during the next five years. For example:

   • Enhancing reputation in the community

   • Improving patient safety

   • Increasing margins to allow investment in new technology

   Meet with the other groups and share your lists. Identify the items on these lists that the groups hold in common. In addition, identify causal linkages among the issues listed. For example, one could emphasize the positive relationships between error reduction and the reputation of the hospital and between cost containment and financial margins.

   At this point in the PAR Process, focus attention on issues that the groups hold in common rather than debating differences that may exist in the lists.

   Discuss the implications of these overlaps, noting that it is important to break down old ways of relating to the other group if progress is to be made on the issues that all groups agree are important.

4. In your PAR transition teams, please carry out the constructive dialogue process described in detail earlier in this chapter.

- Ensure that pre-meeting preparation is thorough and that expectations are carefully communicated.

- Create ground rules using the examples provided earlier in this chapter as guidelines.

- Exchange information following the agenda suggested earlier in the chapter as a way of enhancing understanding and beginning to bridge costly divides between your groups.

A guide from the PCP (Herzig and Chasin 2006) suggests the following sample agenda for such a dialogue:

- Agree on (or review) ground rules.

- Clarify the issue to be the focus of the dialogue.

- First Go-Round (3 minutes each). "Is there something you'd be willing to share about your life experiences that might help others understand your thoughts and feelings about the issue?"

- Second Go-Round (2 minutes each). "As you think about the general perspectives you hold, what's at the heart of the matter for you?"

- Third Go-Round (3 minutes each). "Please speak about any value conflicts, gray areas, or uncertainties you've experienced as you've thought about the issues. For example, perhaps you can think of a time when the values related to this issue that you hold dear bumped up against other values that are also important to you, or a time when you felt yourself pulled in two directions."

- Complete the dialogue by having each participant
  - note a point of learning,
  - pick up and weave a thread or theme from the dialogue, and
  - clarify the differences that remain.

5. Have the transition teams identify initiatives (small wins) that physician and administrative leaders can work on together. Make sure the initiatives

- are doable,

- provide desired benefits for both physicians and administrators,

- have short time frames for early wins, and

- have clear expectations about
  - how to measure success,
  - how to assign ownership and accountability to joint physician and administrative leaders, and
  - how and when results will be reported.

Begin several of these projects simultaneously, recognizing that achieving some positive outcomes is important and that all of the projects may not be successful.

CHAPTER 7

Phase Three: Strengthen Separate Group Security

Disentangled Negative Connections at Louis Martin Community Hospital
Desperate for a solution to the problems plaguing the hospital and sensing the readiness of most administrators and physicians at LMCH to begin relating differently to one another, Mr. Mosher, the CEO, had called us back to reengage them in the process of disentangling the negative connections that had locked the groups in battle.

Transition teams from the medical staff, administration, and board had agreed to begin the work of "untying the knot." Eventually it was possible to engage them in small wins projects, the results of which others at LMCH began to notice. For example, one of the physicians and an administrative leader had jointly established new supervisory practices on one of the floors. They developed clear measures of success in clinical and financial outcomes, and news of their successes traveled throughout the hospital. As a result, physicians and administrators who had remained uninvolved in the PAR Process stepped forward with greater readiness to begin the work of disentanglement through dialogues and a continued series of small wins projects.

Though everyone seemed pleased that the negative charge between the groups throughout LMCH had begun to dissipate, this created another challenge: Each group had lost the glue that had held it together as a distinct unit.

(Continued on following page)

(Continued from previous page)

Without a common enemy, each group became fragmented. So although the joint physician–administrator small wins of the past six months had demonstrated to everyone at LMCH that a different way of relating to one another was possible, cohesion among members of both groups was insufficient to allow either side to envision (much less act upon) a dream of what might ultimately be possible if they came together collaboratively with their peers. Individuals from both sides seemed not even remotely aware of their own group's value and unique contributions to LMCH.

PURPOSE OF THE THIRD PHASE

THE PURPOSE OF the third phase of the PAR Process is to develop satisfaction, pride, and a sense of belonging within each group, and to create among each group's members a sense of security about their group's value and unique contributions to the health system. If physicians feel secure in their group's own distinctive value, they feel less threatened by the strength and successes of administrators, and vice versa. This allows them to remain disentangled from the earlier negative connections between the groups, and it opens up the possibility for each group to envision its respective clinical and administrative dreams.

The group security required to minimize feeling that one's own distinctiveness is threatened is a prerequisite for harmony between groups with fundamental differences (Hornsey and Hogg 2000a). Collaboration between physicians and administrators therefore necessitates maintaining and strengthening each group's sense of its own unique and distinctive contributions, rather than playing down the differences between the groups.

WHY IT IS IMPORTANT

Although administrators and physicians are often considered two groups within healthcare organizations, in reality they are fragmented.

On one side, administrators determine the management of health systems and its acceptance and support in their communities. They are responsible for the business end of healthcare and for the coordination of employees delivering services to their communities. Despite the seeming coherence of their job descriptions, multiple vice presidents and managers at various levels of the organization often work independently and at cross-purposes with one another (Daft 1998). So even though outsiders may view hospital administration as a unified whole, those in administrative positions rarely see themselves this way. Especially when administrators are no longer anchored against the negative "other," there may be little to unite them as a unique and distinctive group.

On the other side, physicians determine appropriate care and ensure that individual patients receive the best care available. Although they are the primary professionals licensed to practice medicine, their collective voice has often remained muted (Reece 2008), and they have not tended to band together as a group except in their animosity toward administrators. With that animosity removed, physicians often find themselves isolated from each other (and from the healthcare organizations at which they practice) (Stubblefield 2005). So here, too, even though outsiders may view physicians as a unified group, this is not how physicians tend to see themselves.

What this means is that in the case of hospital administrators and physicians, there are not just two groups, but multiple fragmented subgroups within each. This is especially true when the common enemy has been removed. The third phase of the PAR Process strengthens the bonds among these fragmented subgroups to develop a strong and secure common identity within each of the groups.

Why go through all this? There are at least two reasons. First, we know that when individuals feel secure in their sense of belonging to a group, they will have greater commitment to the group and to its purpose, they will exhibit more cooperative behaviors (e.g., sit on voluntary committee task forces), and they will demonstrate more citizenship behaviors (e.g., refer patients to other physicians in the system) (Dukerich, Golden, and Shortell 2002). Although common wisdom suggests that people behave primarily according to their self-interests (e.g., resources obtained, sanctions, incentives), research has documented that people's sense of pride in belonging to a distinctive and valued group largely determines their commitment to and their behaviors in that group. A strong sense of belonging even influences people's ability to follow through on failing group-related tasks that they might otherwise abandon (Haslam et al. 2006). One research study (Tyler and Blader 2000) compared self-interest-based costs and benefits (e.g., money) with group membership (peer respect) in terms of predicting certain behaviors. The results indicate that although self-interest-based costs and benefits are important to people, what counts as a cost or as a benefit cannot be established apart from the group memberships that give it meaning (e.g., the resources obtained connote status and respect in one's group). Edwin French (2008), CEO of MedCath in Charlotte, North Carolina, has expressed a similar view of what motivates physicians. In his words, "what physicians want is respect and participation. They want to be heard. These factors transcend economics. Money is a vehicle by which physicians seek what they really want."

The second reason for going through all this is that strong partners make good partners. A group's strong and secure sense of self decreases defensiveness and leads to greater support for efforts that cut across groups. We are beginning to see evidence of this in healthcare. For example, one study surveyed 326 senior physician executives at hospitals and health systems to assess their view of the hospital–physician relationships at their institutions (Bard et al. 2002). The authors found that the level of medical staff group cohesion correlated positively with the level of physician support for organization-wide initiatives and with the success of physician–hospital relationships. That is, the more secure physicians felt about themselves as a distinctive group, the better their relationships were with their hospital system.

Social science research has produced similar findings in various settings. Two groups with very different values will most readily support a common overarching purpose when each group already feels secure, distinctive, and nonthreatened. When only the common purpose is emphasized, deemphasizing and thus threatening the separate group distinctiveness of either group, defensive reactions of turfism and tribalism are likely. For example, one study showed that when ethnic subgroup members of a multiethnic high school experienced their subgroups as highly distinct and secure, this condition produced more positive intergroup relations among people playing on the same team than did a singular focus on the team as a whole (Gaertner and Dovidio 2000). According to this research, only if the separate and distinctive groups are strong and secure about their unique contributions will their members enthusiastically support a common cause.

WHAT IT ENTAILS

Unfortunately, physician and administrative groups have lost much of their sense of (and pride in) who they are as distinct and unique groups. In theory, administrative teams would seem more likely to be unified than medical staffs. This is because the administrative side of hospitals and health systems is thought to be a relatively hierarchical group jointly responsible for coordinating the organization's activities. Because the hierarchy dictates who reports to whom, it seems ideal for coordinating the many people within it, and therefore should lead to a sense of overall group unity. In simple organizations, such as small start-ups, this is probably the case, since one or a few people perform most of the organization's tasks. In complex organizations, such as most health systems, the division of labor is high. The resulting structural silos have created barriers for administrators to seeing one another as belonging to the same team. Beginning in the 1950s, hospitals were organized around functions such as marketing, finance, nursing, and human resources. These functional silos have created areas of specialty that often compete for resources while pursuing separate objectives. More recently, some hospitals have adopted service-line structures that organize specialties around those who need to work together to serve a particular customer need (e.g., cardiology). Of course, while such service-line structures arguably serve the customer more effectively, this has simply created another form of splintering administrative units.

The fragmentation may be even more extreme for physician groups. The specialization, subspecialization, and sub-subspecialization in U.S. medicine over the past decades have fractured the profession into competing subgroups. The medical staff as a negative force is quite powerful, able to block undesirable administrative initiatives very effectively. As a positive force, however, the medical staff is often disorganized, splintered, impotent, and reactive, and it generally only comes together in response to a perceived threat (Bujak 2003). Physicians tend to be individualistic and to see groups as a necessary evil for coping with some of the changes in healthcare. As Bujak (2008) noted in *Inside the Physician Mind*, physicians are taught that they individually bear the ultimate responsibility for their patients; thus they tend to not interfere with what others are doing and to want no interference in return. Most medical staffs are poorly organized; they have no unifying set of values or strategic plan for their group. They are groups in name only. Whatever group culture does exist is often oriented to preserving the existing loose-knit affiliation rather than to developing a stronger physician organization (Bujak 2003; Gillies et al. 2001).

The challenge before physician and administrative leaders, then, is to ensure that each group feels secure about its distinctive and unique contributions before attempting to motivate its members toward a common purpose and to engage the members of each group in behaviors that signal the value and distinctiveness of their own group, before attempting to engage them more fully in system-wide behaviors. Physicians *have* mobilized as a group out of outrage about issues such as a broken Medicare system, against health plans formulating quality rankings and steering patient treatment, and to resist the implementation of new systems (e.g., outcomes measurement and technologies such as electronic medical records). Administrators, too, have mobilized as a group out of anger, frustration, or fear of external threats. To be sure, these forms of mobilization have created a sense of unity, but it is negatively motivated and reactionary. The problem is that this is likely to pull physicians and administrators back into the locked-up state of oppositional entanglement.

A more promising avenue is for members of both groups to mobilize out of a positive sense of who they are. Positive group self-perceptions can derive from connections among peers even beyond the organization. As an example, physicians are starting to realize the power of the Internet to mobilize and transmit information about their professional work with their peers around the world. Relevant websites include the following (Reece 2008):

- Physicians Interactive, which claims to represent more than 500,000 physicians—a leading source of information about medications (PhysiciansInteractive.com);
- DoctorsHangout, a social networking website for medical students and residents (DoctorsHangout.com); and
- Sermo, a physicians-only medical observations networking site that had more than 70,000 participating physicians in 2008 (sermo.com).

Hospital administrators, too, have opportunities to forge greater group connections through membership in associations such as the American College of Healthcare Executives (ACHE), which supports administrators in meeting the best and brightest in the field through the diverse membership of more than 30,000 healthcare leaders from the United States, Canada, and abroad. Frequent national and regional meetings, an online affiliate directory, and message boards give members an easy way to connect. Local chapters also provide networking, education, and career development opportunities. For example, the Eastern Pennsylvania Healthcare Executive Network is an active independent chapter of ACHE. Purposes of this local chapter are

- to promote professional interaction and communication among individuals with responsibility in the administration of healthcare facilities and agencies,

- to promote and foster the advancement of leadership and competency in healthcare management by providing an educational forum for leaders in health-related management fields,
- to address political and economic issues impacting healthcare in the region and the state, and
- to promote networking among its members and professional organizations and to encourage participation in the American College of Healthcare Executives and other appropriate health or professional associations.

Creating peer-to-peer connections of this kind tends to reduce defensiveness and opens up conversations about what the group is already doing, allowing members to build on their capabilities and strengthening group ties. We offer a number of suggestions for strengthening the security of administrative and physician groups beyond forging connections with peers outside the organization. Social science research and healthcare best practice examples provide clear and well-tested prescriptions for encouraging group members to feel strong, secure, and proud of their group membership (Ashforth and Mael 1989; Fiol, Pratt, and O'Connor 2009). Some are self-evident; others are less so.

Identify Commonalities

First, it is important to stress the similar values among members of each group and to promote the development of common visions among group members based on those values. Despite the fragmented subspecialties that create perceptions of differences, your physicians share a concern for patient safety, a struggle for clinical excellence, and a competitive enthusiasm for effective medical advancements. Your administrators share an interest in the financial viability of the organization, its reputation in the community, and its growth aspirations for the future. The commonalities on both sides are too often overlooked or taken for granted. They need to be explicitly highlighted to develop distinctive common visions within each group.

As an example of a physician dream, Kettering Medical Center, a 520-bed hospital in Dayton, Ohio, organized a heart institute with physician leadership among their cardiologists and cardiac surgeons. The common vision of these physician leaders was improved cath lab utilization and case turnaround, technology acquisition, and patient care in the cardiac care unit (Guthrie, Froneberger, and Terry 2005). As an example on the administrative side, the administrators of a community hospital in the Midwest came together to pursue the possibility of becoming a regional medical center with state-of-the-art telemedicine technology, making the hospital the central node in a three-state network. Formerly adversarial in protecting their turf, the information technology specialists now partnered with financial and marketing experts to articulate the administrative team's new dream.

Formally Articulate Each Group's Priorities

Second, we recommend formally articulating the priorities of each group. For example, a medical advisory panel (MAP) (Cohn, Gill, and Schwartz 2005), used by a number of organizations around the country, may be charged with determining and articulating a hospital's clinical priorities. It solicits systematic input from the medical staff through a series of meetings with each clinical department about opportunities for improvement in patient care and reductions in the hassle for physicians. For example, a 350-bed community teaching hospital in the northeastern United States, plagued by financial losses and troubled relations between physicians and hospital management, convened a MAP charged with determining and articulating the hospital's clinical priorities for the upcoming three years. The panel members were selected based on their clinical ability, leadership skills, and peer credibility. Those involved agreed that the process offered physicians (salaried and independent) the opportunity to share common aspirations and to bond as a group (Cohn, Gill, and Schwartz 2005).

Although a MAP is a useful tool for uniting physicians as a group, clients have expressed concerns that the MAP process focuses solely on physicians, without a parallel attempt to develop connections among hospital administrators. We strongly recommend that a second MAP (*management* advisory panel) be established that performs the same functions for administrative teams. To reiterate, when *both* clinical and administrative groups feel secure in their own unique and distinctive contributions, there is a much better chance for establishing collaboration between them.

Highlight the Attractiveness of Belonging to Each Group

Third, it is important to find ways to highlight the attractiveness of belonging to each of the groups in your system. Although granting benefits along with group membership undoubtedly enhances the attractiveness of belonging to a group, clearly and consistently communicating the prestige and value of each group may contribute to the same end. You might demonstrate respect by routinely including positive patient care stories and statistics in a newsletter, or you might publicly emphasize the administrative team's success in creating a beautiful new facility. Such news releases and the excitement they communicate about the excellence of each group's work give the members a sense of pride in being part of a prestigious group.

Publicize Group Membership

A related approach is to find ways to make membership in each group highly visible across the perceived boundaries that separate the different subgroups and across the community as a whole. This can be done through newsletters, announcements, flyers, push e-mail, or other forms of communication to and about the group. For example, the efforts of leaders implementing the administrative dream of transforming a community hospital into the center of a three-state network were publicized in mailings and newspaper articles across the area. Similarly, a 400-bed, two-hospital system in the West began a promotional program in the community that featured key physician leaders in the two cardiology groups that accounted for 90 percent of their inpatient cardiology care. These examples are public and visible demonstrations of respect for the unique value and distinctive contributions of administrator and physician groups, respectively.

Develop a Measurement System

Finally, it is important to develop a clear measurement system to monitor the value created by each group and to establish performance management systems that are relevant to those outcomes. Administrative performance measurement systems already exist in most healthcare systems (e.g., efficiency, liquidity, growth measures), though you may wish to alter them to better reflect the outcomes of the entire group. Although data on physician performance may be routinely collected and fed back to physicians, often little is done with the information. One study found that the physicians interviewed indicated that they and their colleagues looked at performance results, but felt no need to change the way they practiced as a result (Gillies et al. 2001). If the performance management system is developed for and by the physician leaders—rather than by the administration—and focused on issues critical to physicians, physicians are more likely to be interested in the outcomes. Physicians care about things that waste their time, make them wait, and treat them as a commodity. Leaders of successful programs are more likely to work with their physicians to identify metrics related to these concerns and to regularly monitor and publish information about progress. Such metrics may include turnaround time in the operating room, delays in administering medications, scheduling delays, medical errors, public perception information, and various clinical markers.

Regardless which of approach you implement at your organization, the key is to continue to enhance and promote the image of each group as valuable and unique. Efforts to promote the unity and strength of physicians as a group are already occurring (Advisory Board Company 2007). For example, 50 physicians in Boston-based Beth Israel Deaconess Medical Center's cardiology, cardiac surgery, and vascular surgery departments formed the Cardiovascular Institute, a corporation that promotes interdisciplinary cooperation and allows physicians to draft treatment protocols (e.g., which specialists can implant stents) to decrease the potential for conflicts among the specialists. Such collaboration aims to enable physicians to choose the best treatment for patients, rather than just doing what she or he does best. Similarly, in 2006, physicians at Massachusetts General Hospital established a vascular center in Boston and Waltham that encompassed seven specialties, all of which agreed to advertise only collectively. Here too, the group determines which physicians perform certain procedures based on criteria they have developed in common. Physicians associated with Brigham and Women's Hospital have been negotiating agreements among various specialties that will allow patients to see multiple specialists during a single visit and to receive a collaborative treatment recommendation and a single bill. And Baptist Health Care in Pensacola, Florida, has created physician loyalty teams, whose job it is to determine the primary irritants for their physicians and to turn those situations into positive "WOW! Events" (Stubblefield 2005). What if your healthcare organization created physician and administrator loyalty teams?

WHY IT IS LIKELY TO BE RESISTED

Past experience has taught most physicians and administrators that strengthening and unifying the other group poses a very real threat. Why would you want the "other" to develop a strong and unified sense of group pride when the only thing that has held your own group together in the past is the common threat of "them" taking away your autonomy and interfering with your work? The idea that the other group may become even stronger is often a scary one.

Even the unification of one's own group may be resisted, given the competitive nature that often characterizes administrative functions and medical subspecialties. An example of the resistance to unite on the physician side is the failed attempt to unionize. In 1999, the American Medical Association (AMA) approved a national union for employed physicians to help them negotiate better terms with their hospitals and to level the playing field with powerful managed care organizations. The AMA abandoned the union in 2004 after spending at least $3.6 million on the venture, which organized only 38 physicians in four years—a cost of about $95,000 per physician. AMA officials said little about the reason for the failure of this costly plan (Romano 2004a), but it does reflect the difficulty of mobilizing physicians as a group.

HOW TO MOVE THROUGH THE RESISTANCE

Group Leadership

Effective leadership on both sides is critical for moving through the resistance. The key is to convincingly convey the notion that each group's security in its own unique distinctiveness actually makes each group less, rather than more, threatening. Leaders need not hold formal positions in the organization to be convincing, but they need to be credible (which is why we argued in Chapter 4 that the most important criterion for transition team membership is credibility). Significant research suggests that one of the most important leadership attributes to gain member endorsement is that the leader be prototypical of the group—that is, that he or she represent the interests and characteristics of the group. People are more likely to trust members of their own group and by extension are more likely to trust leaders who are seen as credible members of their own group. In fact, researchers have found that perceptions of the leader as "one of us" are more important for leader endorsement than are perceptions that the leader is "doing it for us." So even if leaders appear to be allocating resources unfairly (not "doing it for us"), they are more likely to be supported if people perceive them as "one of us" (Haslam and Platow 2001).

On the surface, it would seem that such leadership is readily available on both sides. The hierarchical structure of most administrative departments provides a framework for the unification of administrators as a group. The challenge is to identify leaders who really are perceived by all or most administrators as part of "us." If the chief financial officer of the hospital, for example, is perceived as being part of the finance team, but not supportive of the rest of the administrative group, she would not be a wise choice to lead this security-building process.

Such leadership also seems to be available on the physician side. Physician executives are growing in number and influence in U.S. healthcare. Healthcare futurist Russell Coile stated that 15,000 physicians were taking top jobs in leading hospitals, health systems, and medical groups across the nation (Casanova 2004). But moving into an executive position often means that physicians must depart from their solely clinical sense of self. They often begin to define themselves—and others begin to define them—as business executives who happen to be doctors. Such physician executives are sometimes more focused on administrative concerns than on strengthening and uniting physicians as a group. A focus on physicians and their concerns is essential to building a strong, distinctive, and secure physician group.

Focus Group Members on Themselves

An effective way to move through the inevitable resistance is to continue focusing the members of each group on themselves, rather than on the "other." If people are focused on what makes their group distinctive, valuable, and unique, they are less likely to be threatened by the strength of the "other." Therefore, a focus on building the security of one's own group is likely to ultimately lead to better partnerships with the other. What can we learn about this from corporate alliances, which have to manage entities that often have opposing cultures and operating procedures? Corporate alliances have been tremendously popular recently, soaring 25 percent a year. Yet the failure rate is around 70 percent. According to Fred Hassan, the CEO of Schering-Plough in 2007, "Alliances require ways of working with partners that are very different from what is required in traditional business relationships. The future will belong to those companies that embed alliance management capabilities into the fabric of their culture" (Hughes and Weiss 2007, 9).

One of the key principles for effective corporate alliances may serve as a lesson here: Spend as much time managing internal stakeholders as you do managing the relationship with the partner. Conventional advice—to serve the partnership at all costs—may be bad advice. In fact, in focusing on the partnership, one often loses commitment from and alignment among the units and functions of one's own group (i.e., physician leaders lose alignment among the various aspects of the clinical delivery system, and administrators lose alignment among the various aspects of the management system). For example, in the late 1990s two financial services companies formed an alliance to exploit technological developments enabling electronic payments (Hughes and Weiss 2007). They devoted a great deal of time and effort to learning about one another and to managing their interactions. In fact, they worked very well together. But as they focused increasingly on how they should work together, they lost control of what was happening within their own organizations. Fragmentation within each organization eventually made it impossible to coordinate effectively with the partner. Some reported that they felt as if they were managing an alliance with multiple partners rather than one. For this reason, ongoing management of one's own unit is an essential part of making an alliance work.

Identify the Benefits That Arise from Differences

Another way to reduce resistance to building strong and secure groups is to identify the benefits that can arise from the differences between groups. We can again learn from the experience of corporate alliances. One of the key principles for managing such alliances is to leverage the differences of alliance partners to create value rather than trying to eliminate them. A common refrain goes something like this (Hughes and Weiss 2007, 5): "Our differences are slowing us down. Let's just figure out one way of getting things done and move on." Of course, what this usually means is, "You need to accept *our* way of doing things." These efforts send a message that differences are bad. They drive the conflict underground (but not for long), and they erode people's ability to make use of the very differences that could make the combined organization successful.

The alliance between Hewlett-Packard (HP) and Microsoft, under which HP hosted Microsoft's Exchange messaging and collaboration software at its data centers, is an example. The companies had different but complementary strengths in technical expertise, culture, and knowledge of the market. Despite a lot of work at the outset of the alliance to clearly define the larger unit's goals and rules of engagement between the partners, each side began to see the other as incompetent, untrustworthy, or downright crazy. The relationship deteriorated until the companies began to systematically document differences between the partners and then met to discuss how those differences were being perceived and whether they might actually benefit the alliance. Eventually, their frustrations with one another exploded, and their perceptions of each other poured out in highly inflammatory language. As the story goes (Hughes and Weiss 2007), once the air was cleared and the differences were discussed in a productive way, each side was able to see some of its own weaknesses and some of its partner's strengths. Ultimately, they were able to actively leverage the differences.

DISSEMINATION OF SEPARATE GROUP SECURITY BEYOND OPINION LEADERS

Physicians and administrators may initially have little interest in strengthening the bonds among their peers. As in the earlier phases, we recommend that you begin the process by drawing on the physician and administrator champions in the innovator/opinion leader transition teams, engaging them in establishing a common vision and a tentative set of common priorities within each of their own peer groups. The tentative priorities can then be used to recruit their peers and to revise and refine their common group vision. Your board plays an essential role in championing the distinctive value and contributions of the physician and administrative groups at your hospital and in overseeing the process each group undertakes to strengthen its separate security.

CHAPTER SUMMARY

When interdependent groups are fundamentally different, each must be secure in its own distinctive value before it can sustain a collaborative relationship with the other. Chapter 7 described the processes for strengthening physician and administrative groups and for enhancing each group's security about the value of its unique contributions to the overall system. After noting the purpose of the phase and why it is important, we provided specific approaches you may adopt to apply this phase in your organization. The assessment exercises at the end of this chapter will give you a sense of the fragmentation of groups in your organization and their need to be unified around their unique value, and the exercises for promoting separate group security summarize the steps for achieving this outcome. Only when the members of each group feel a sense of pride, belonging, and security about their own group does it make sense to begin to develop *separate togetherness*, which we turn to in Chapter 8.

SELF-ASSESSMENT EXERCISES

Assessing the Security of Groups at Your Organization

Please respond to each statement in Sections 1 and 2 by indicating your level of agreement on a scale ranging from Strongly Disagree (1) to Strongly Agree (5).

Depending on who is completing the assessment, Section 1 will provide information about how physicians actually view the security of their group, *or* administrators' and trustees' opinions about the security of physicians as a group. Similarly, Section 2 will provide information about how administrators actually view the security of their group, *or* physicians' and trustees' opinions about the security of administrators as a group.

Section 1: Physicians

Physicians have a well-articulated clinical vision that clarifies outcomes that are important to the majority of the medical staff. _____

Physicians feel secure about the distinctive contributions of their group. _____

Physicians recognize the potential value of administrators, even if bitter disagreements remain. _____

Physicians are willing to employ decision-making methods that include administrators' preferred styles (e.g., time used, degree of discussion, etc.). _____

Physicians are proud of measured outcomes that document their valued contributions. _____

Physicians talk about being valuable because of the contribution they make, not because they are different (better) than administrators. _____

Physicians think of the medical staff's successes as
their own successes.   _____

Average score for Section 1   _____

Section 2: Administrators

Administrators have a well-articulated managerial
vision that clarifies outcomes that are important to
the majority of administrators.   _____

Administrators feel secure about the distinctive contributions of their group.   _____

Administrators recognize the potential value of physicians, even if bitter disagreements remain.   _____

Administrators are willing to employ decision-making
methods that include physicians' preferred styles (e.g.,
time used, degree of discussion).   _____

Administrators are proud of measured outcomes that
document their valued contributions.   _____

Administrators talk about being valuable because of
the contribution they make, not because they are
different (better) than physicians.   _____

Administrators think of the administrative team's
successes as their own successes.   _____

Average score for Section 2   _____

Please average the scores for Section 1 and Section 2 separately.

If you are a physician, the average score of Section 1 reveals how
you view the security of your own group; if you are an administrator

or board member, the average score in Section 1 reveals your opinions about the security of physicians as a group.

If you are an administrator, the average score of Section 2 reveals how you view the security of your own group; if you are a physician or board member, the average score in Section 2 reveals your opinions about the security of administrators as a group.

How do the groups at your organization look when evaluated against these statements? High average scores indicate that your organization may have done the work required to develop physician and administrative groups that are secure about their unique and distinctive contributions. However, any average score below four (4) suggests the need for serious consideration, if not further action to strengthen security within the groups. What changes would be helpful to develop more secure physician and administrative groups?

EXERCISES FOR PROMOTING GROUP SECURITY

If people are highly resistant to the promotion of each group's security, we suggest beginning with the following steps:

1. Ensure that each PAR Process transition team has one or more credible leaders (formal or informal) who can convincingly persuade their peers that the other group's security in its own distinctive contributions will make it less, rather than more, threatening to their group.

   To strengthen their persuasion, leaders can draw upon lessons they learned in Phase Two of the PAR Process. For example, they might remind their peers that

   • the groups share many common interests;

   • a number of small wins initiatives jointly undertaken by physicians and administrators are already underway, the most successful of which tend to be the result of strong partners (rather than weak or dominated partners); and

   • secure groups are more likely to exhibit cooperative than defensive behaviors.

2. Continue to focus the members of each group on their own distinctive contributions to avoid slippage back into security based on opposition to the other group.

3. Identify the potential benefits that arise from differences between the groups.

   • Systematically document each group's different styles and capabilities.

- Discuss how those differences are currently perceived.

- Explore which of the differences might benefit everyone involved and what that would require.

- Identify specific strategies for actively promoting and leveraging those differences.

As resistance lessens and people become more aware of the benefits of each group feeling secure about its own unique contributions, they may be ready to engage in the following exercises for further promoting group security.

4. Collect information on physician and administrator associations and networks that promote contact among their members.

Actively promote involvement in these associations and networks, with periodic assessments to ensure that the involvement is leading to greater security regarding the value contributed by people's own peer groups rather than perpetuating old conversations about what is wrong with the "other."

5. Develop a medical staff vision based on values the physicians hold in common and a management vision based on values the administrators hold in common.

Sponsor physician-only and administrator-only retreats for each group to develop its vision.

Questions to ask include:

- What is our physician dream? Or what is our administrative dream?

- What do we value most, no matter what?

- What do we really want to accomplish?

- What are we the best at?

- What are we proudest of?

6. Formally articulate the priorities of each group.

  - Form a medical advisory panel to determine and articulate your hospital's clinical priorities and values.

  - Form a management advisory panel to determine and articulate your hospital's administrative priorities and values.

The following steps may be useful in both forming advisory panels and developing the priorities:

  - Clarify the process for the board and seek their support.

  - Select panel leaders based on their credibility among peers and leadership skills.

  - Provide the time, information, and technical skills required for success.

  - Collect verbal and written information about the priorities each department views as essential to success.

  - Prioritize recommendations within each of the panels based on their broad positive impact on the overall delivery of care now and in the future.

  - Compile a written report of recommendations that is broadly supported by your peers.

  - Present priority recommendations to the hospital board.

7. Identify the benefits of being a member of a very successful physician team. Highlight these benefits in discussions with members of the medical staff.

Examples of benefits to highlight might include the following:

- The autonomy to focus on clinical versus administrative tasks

- The resources needed to acquire physical facilities, technologies, and staff to provide state-of-the-art patient treatments

- Recognition as the team that created effective physician–administrator collaboration

8. Identify the benefits of being a member of a very successful administrative team. Highlight these benefits in discussions among administrators.

Examples of benefits to highlight might include the following:

- Being sought out by healthcare leaders coming to learn how productive physician–administrator team performance can be achieved

- Enjoying market domination by being able to
  - avoid the distractions of physician–administrator conflicts and
  - successfully focus on managing resources to achieve your vision

- Being the beneficiary of new revenue streams, such as
  - visitation fees from healthcare leaders who come to observe your successful system and

- consulting fees from requested interventions at other healthcare organizations

- Enjoying personal benefits of success including

    - speaking invitations to share your success story with other healthcare leaders and

    - job offers to implement similar successes

9. Make membership in each group highly visible across your entire community by publicizing the distinctive contributions of physicians and administrators. Use a variety of media to get the word out, including

- newsletters,

- announcements,

- flyers,

- push e-mail,

- press releases,

- newspaper articles,

- celebrations, and

- website recognition.

10. Develop a clear measurement system to document the value created by each group.

Questions to ask include the following:

- What is already working in our situation, or what success are we currently having? What makes it work, or what causes our success?

- What outcome data do we need to collect to demon-strate our progress toward our dream?

- How should we report the data in order to interest our peers in what we are doing?

CHAPTER 8

Phase Four: Promote Separate Togetherness

The most difficult problem of all is to unite voice and instruments so they blend in the rhythmic motion of a piece and the instruments support and enhance the voice in its emotional expression, for voices and instruments are by their nature opposed to each other …

—Josiah Fisk, *Composers on Music: Eight Centuries of Writings*, 1956

Strong and Secure Separate Groups at Louis Martin Community Hospital

The energy and morale at Louis Martin Community Hospital were higher than they had been for as long as people could remember. Physicians were spending more time at the hospital and more time with each other. Three months ago, the physician transition team in collaboration with Dr. Schmidt had organized a medical staff retreat, which was well attended. At the retreat, the medical staff developed a preliminary description of what great patient care would look like at LMCH. It also elected a medical advisory panel consisting of seven respected

(Continued on following page)

(Continued from previous page)

and credible physicians, whose charge it was to collect information from their peers and formally articulate the medical priorities. The priorities were developed and circulated among all of the medical staff, and buy-in was strong.

The growing strength and security of the physicians as a united group was something no one had ever witnessed at LMCH. Initially, senior administrators at the hospital saw this as a threat. In fact, Mr. Mosher, the CEO, remembering the former attempts of the medical staff to oust him, approached us with concerns about what this would mean for his position and for the hospital's viability in the future. We took this as an opportunity to reiterate the benefits to all involved when both groups are strengthened and given more, rather than less, autonomy and authority.

Within weeks, the administrative transition team in collaboration with Mr. Mosher had mobilized the administrators to follow a process similar to the one the physicians had gone through. They formed a management advisory panel consisting of administrators from different functional areas of the hospital to generate administrative priorities that would broadly reflect the interests of the entire group.

LMCH board members had uniformly supported the earlier processes of promoting readiness to begin the PAR Process, and they had been especially pleased with the way the disentangling process had reduced the tensions that had long been paralyzing everyone at the hospital. The passion with which physicians and administrators were now articulating their dreams and priorities further ignited board members' excitement and enthusiasm. They publicly announced the merits and accomplishments of each group, ensuring that the community surrounding the hospital was aware of these diverse contributions. Of course, this made group members even more secure and even clearer about the benefits of belonging to their group.

The energy was palpable, the enthusiasm contagious. But work still needed to be done to ensure sustained collaboration between physicians and administrators at LMCH.

PURPOSE OF THE FOURTH PHASE

THE PURPOSE OF the fourth and final phase of the PAR Process is to align the members of each group (i.e., physicians, administrators, and trustees) around a joint purpose without sacrificing the separate strength and security of their own groups. The separate group security achieved in Phase Three is not, by itself, sufficient. Physicians and administrators are highly interdependent and cannot isolate themselves from one another. In international politics, the dimensions that determine interdependence are sensitivity and vulnerability (Keohane and Nye 1977). Sensitivity is the extent to which one party (e.g., physicians) is affected by the actions of another (e.g., administrators); vulnerability is the inability of a party to insulate itself from those effects. Interdependence is a condition in which each party is highly sensitive and vulnerable in its relationship with the other. In healthcare, physicians and administrators are certainly interdependent along those two dimensions, which suggests that each group needs the other to accomplish its goals. The groups therefore must come together while remaining secure in their separateness.

Evidence from social science research and experience in healthcare indicate that this is possible *if* each group is secure in its own unique distinctiveness before attempts to bring the groups together are initiated. In Chapter 3, we described a study of multiple ethnic groups all playing on the same team. The study found that playing down ethnic differences and highlighting the collective team identity was associated with greater bias and conflict among the groups (Gaertner and Dovidio 2000). The same study found that the least intergroup bias and conflict occurred when students perceived themselves as unique and separate along ethnic lines and united in playing on the same team. We refer to this as *separate togetherness*: Groups see themselves as distinct and *separate* from the "other," while at the same time they work *together* with that "other" toward a common purpose (Fiol, Pratt, and O'Connor 2009; Gaertner and Dovidio 2000; Gaertner et al. 1999). Promoting simultaneous separateness and togetherness is the purpose of the fourth phase of the PAR Process.

WHY IT IS IMPORTANT

Promoting the separate togetherness of physicians and administrators at your hospital is important for at least two reasons. First, attempts to promote togetherness alone are likely to be resisted. In Chapter 3, we described why efforts to unite physicians and hospital administrators in support of a common vision have proven to be so difficult. These groups have distinct, often conflicting perspectives on who they are and what is most important. Their knowledge bases, backgrounds, education, and priorities all point in different directions. Attempts to emphasize that "we're all in this together" have not proven successful in most cases (Budetti et al. 2002), because the groups tend to respond by defensively proving their distinctiveness. It is easier for people to buy into and develop their connections within the larger unit when they do not have to defend their own group's distinctiveness. Only if the separate distinctiveness of each group is strong and secure are members likely to support the larger unit.

Second, attempts to promote separateness alone are likely to fail. A health system needs both groups to work together to produce the desired results. This seems obvious, considering administrators' need for physicians to deliver healthcare. The reverse is usually true as well. Physicians need the skills that administrators bring to the table, even though they may sometimes lose sight of this, as exemplified by the rise and fall of a physician-owned hospital in Denver, Colorado. In early 1998, a group of Denver physicians invested their personal resources and millions of borrowed dollars to develop Precedent Health Center. According to one of the executives, the physician ownership and management of the hospital put doctors on the road to regaining control of healthcare (Algeo 1997). Excellence in patient care and service was the vision, and investments were made to achieve it: Amenities included private suites with personal chefs, free day care for outpatients' children, a state-of-the-art digital radiology department, and a staff large enough to provide one-on-one care—in short, a physician's dream. Despite its investments in excellent clinical care and service, the hospital suffered from cash-flow problems, it did not land the insurance contracts it had hoped for, its billing and phone systems were not up to par, and overhead costs were high and rising (Conklin 1998). After hemorrhaging red ink throughout its 14-month life, Precedent closed its doors. The lack of management expertise was cited as a major reason for the failure of the venture (Hubler 1999). The example illustrates our point: The expertise of both physicians and administrators is essential to the success of healthcare organizations.

WHAT IT ENTAILS

Separate togetherness will not happen by itself. Leaders must foster the conditions that support its development and continue to nurture these conditions over time. The key is to develop "us *and* them" versus "us *or* them" thinking. Historically, "or" thinking has dominated in healthcare. For example, a physician-to-physician satisfaction study conducted by the Center for Health Futures at Florida Hospital in Orlando found that hospital cost-containment efforts topped the list as the source of *least* satisfaction for physicians; of course, these efforts are of *most* concern to administrators (Bogue et al. 2006).

By contrast, separate togetherness implies that each group needs the other to win for its own group to win. For example, a West Coast teaching hospital had tried unsuccessfully to reduce the number of joint replacement implant vendors. Vendors bypassed hospital administrators, leaving the hospital to pay the difference between implant cost and Medicare reimbursement. Recognizing the potential benefits of "and" thinking, orthopedic surgeons at the hospital convinced their peers to standardize processes and consolidate vendors. All but one surgeon agreed to a single vendor and a unified operative approach, which saved the hospital more than $4 million over three years. This reduction in the diversity of implants used had no effect on clinical outcomes. The hospital reinvested about $365,000 of the savings in updated operating room equipment, which was the only purchase that the orthopedic surgeons requested

(Cohn and Allyn 2005). This is an example of win–win "and" versus "or" thinking. We have found the following strategies and tactics useful for developing such thinking.

Develop a Statement of Purpose for the Larger Unit That Requires Each Group's Separate Distinctive Contributions

Ensuring that your physician and administrative groups feel strong, distinctive, secure, and nonthreatened and igniting pride in belonging to such a group are the first steps toward healing the broken relations between hospitals and physicians. Understanding and explicitly articulating the priorities and contributions of each group set the stage for identifying a larger purpose that encompasses their multiple interests. What is the overarching purpose that can draw your physicians and administrators together, while at the same time allowing them to retain pride and satisfaction in their separate and distinctive contributions?

When developing your statement of purpose, it is important to focus equally on the possibilities of the health system as a whole and the interests of the separate groups. An analogy for this approach is fusion cooking, which combines different ethnic foods and cooking techniques into one dish, while preserving their distinct cultural flavors, textures, and presentations. Fusion cooking has four principles:

- Respect the different ingredients.
- Recognize the value of combining the different ingredients.
- Set a goal of creative but realistic dishes.
- Preserve the identity of cultural ingredients in those dishes.

Fusion is not just a cooking technique. This approach is getting serious attention from political scientists and government officials dealing with multicultural populations who are resisting full integration or assimilation, preferring to protect their unique cultures

(Brett and Janssens 2006). What would the four fusion cooking principles look like when applied to your health system? Too often, physicians invest time and energy in trying to convince administrators or payers of the need to spend more to meet a specific patient's clinical needs, and too often administrators argue that physicians should be more interested in the long-term financial well-being of their health system. These approaches seldom produce enduring success. Rather than attempting to convince the "other" to be more like you, collaboration is more likely to result from (1) respecting the groups' different skills, (2) recognizing the value of combining those skills, (3) developing a creative but realistic statement of purpose, and (4) preserving the identity of both groups as they align around that purpose. These are the four underlying principles of separate togetherness.

Leo Bressanelli, CEO of Genesis Health Systems in Davenport, Iowa, described an example of physician–hospital separate togetherness. The health system and the area's largest group of cardiologists collaborated to create the Genesis Heart Institute. Physicians offered diagnostic testing services, and across the skywalk from their offices, the hospital offered rehabilitation services. Bressanelli noted that it is "somewhat unique to have those centers side by side. One is an extension of the physicians' offices and one is an extension of the hospital's services." The institute was governed by a board of directors composed of an equal number of physicians and health system executives (Haugh 2005).

Following the principles of separate togetherness in developing a statement of purpose for your organization will allow you to identify performance outcomes that require the distinctive inputs of the different groups. Such a purpose increases the likelihood of achieving true coequal partnership among the groups. As an example, Louis Martin Community Hospital developed the following purpose statement: "Best place to give and get care, now and in the future." Administrators, physicians, and trustees at LMCH could all fully align with the purpose, make it their own, and see how it required each of their group's unique contributions. Focusing on each group's own distinctive contributions to this overarching purpose made it less likely that any group would feel threatened and therefore undermine the collaboration. Creating the "best place to give and get care, now and in the future" provided a mutually meaningful purpose that allowed for distinctive roles for clinical (discover and deliver the best treatments) and administrative (acquire technology, manage resources, market distinctiveness) groups. Allowing each group to draw on its distinctive contributions by addressing issues it finds to be pressing enhances the likelihood of the partnership's success.

Connect the Dots

A unique and distinctive set of roles for each group is important in minimizing old power struggles. But the roles must be coordinated. A recent report of Verispan's annual Top 100 Integrated Health Networks, which ranks organizations with effective coordinating mechanisms that allow them to excel clinically and financially, described top systems such as Covenant Healthcare and Presbyterian Healthcare as improving clinical outcomes and cutting costs by "connecting the dots," coordinating the interests of administrators and clinicians throughout their systems (Colias 2004). While the dots do need to be connected, we would further argue that the connected dots need to remain separate and distinctive.

Coordinating the tasks, functions, and interests of separate subgroups so that they work together instead of at cross purposes has long been a challenge in many industries, and a number of integrating mechanisms have been developed (Galbraith 1973). Table 8.1 summarizes mechanisms that have been successful (in order of increasing complexity) and provides an example of each mechanism as it has been applied to Johnson & Johnson (Jones 2004). Which mechanism is appropriate for your organization depends on a number of factors, including the size and diversity of subgroups in the organization and the complexity of their tasks and functions.

Table 8.1 Integration Mechanisms at Johnson & Johnson

Integration Mechanism	Description	Application at Johnson & Johnson (J&J)
Direct contact	Individuals/groups meet face-to-face to coordinate activities.	Diaper Division sales and manufacturing managers meet to discuss scheduling.
Liaison role	Specific individuals are given responsibility for coordinating with the other on behalf of their own subunit.	A person from each of J&J's production, marketing, and R&D departments is given responsibility for coordinating with the other departments.
Task force	Individuals meet in temporary committees to coordinate cross-functional activities.	A committee is formed to find new ways to recycle diapers.
Team	Individuals meet regularly in permanent committees to coordinate activities.	A permanent J&J committee is established to promote new product development in the Diaper Division.
Integrating role	A new role is established to coordinate the activities of two or more functions or divisions.	One manager takes responsibility for coordinating Diaper and Baby Soap divisions to enhance their marketing activities.
Integrating department	A new department is created to coordinate the activities of functions or divisions.	A team of managers is created to take responsibility for coordinating J&J's centralization program to allow divisions to share skills and resources.

SOURCE: Adapted from Jones (2004).

Rewrite the Old Compacts

Compacts are shared understandings of what people owe one another in organizational settings—what each party gives and gets. When fundamental changes make old compacts unworkable, the compacts must evolve. For decades, the compacts in American industry involved job security in exchange for loyalty and hard work. The need for business to be globally competitive and other environmental, social, and economic changes caused a breakdown in the assumed compacts in the latter part of the twentieth century, which resulted in shock and anger across many industries.

In healthcare, physicians' understanding of what they give has typically included delivering quality care, while the "get" part of their compact with hospitals has included control over care delivery and protection from the hassles of running the business side of healthcare (Silversin and Kornacki 2000). Administrators' understanding of what they give has often included providing excellent facilities, while the "get" part of their compact has been physicians' loyalty to the hospital. These old compacts are becoming obsolete. Although they promote separation of the groups, they do not encourage the active alignment of coequal partners that is needed in today's rapidly changing environment. But just as in other industries, failing to abide by the precepts of the old compacts will result in anger, frustration, and increased distrust between the parties. When obsolete compacts get in the way of needed change, they must be reshaped through a structured and overt process, with buy-in from all sides. The process should uncover the assumed and often unstated give-and-get expectations, decide which elements of the old compacts are counterproductive, and identify new expectations that are more closely aligned with current requirements for the success of all involved (Silversin and Kornacki 2000).

Separate togetherness among your physicians and administrators will require new compacts that reflect the principles of fusion we described earlier. Participants must agree to a time frame and a process for implementation and accountability. Other levers for making new compacts real include policies that are consistent with the new compacts, resource allocations that are aligned with the new compacts, measurement and feedback about the extent to which each group is living up to the new compacts, and some part of the compensation and reward system that is tied to meeting the expectations of the new compacts (Silversin and Kornacki 2000).

Foster New Ways of Thinking and Speaking

Separate togetherness entails a new way of thinking and speaking about "us" and "them." Linguistic experts have provided evidence that you can actually prime the way people think of themselves through the conscious use of reference pronouns. For example, the inclusive pronoun "we" makes people feel that they are part of the reference group even though everyone in the group may be strangers, while "us" and "them" create feelings of territoriality and separateness even when people have no history as opposing groups (Fiol 1989). Reference pronouns like "I," "we," "you," and "they" thus serve as powerful signals of who's in and who's out.

To whom, specifically, are you referring when you use the word "us" in a medical staff meeting? Using such pronouns consciously and strategically is important as you manage the boundaries between separate and distinct groups and your health system as a whole. When addressing the medical staff about their concerns as a separate group, "us" should explicitly refer to the medical staff, and "them" should refer to nonmedical staff, reinforcing the distinctiveness of the clinicians as a group. In contrast, when the focus of the communication is the entire health system, "us" should explicitly refer to the system as a whole, with "them" referring to outsiders, such as the system's competitors in the marketplace (Fiol 1989; Fiol, Pratt, and O'Connor 2009).

Foster New Ways of Behaving

Language is a powerful tool. But you cannot sustain people's simultaneous sense of themselves as members of a distinctive and separate group and as members of a common larger unit unless the language is consistent with your behaviors. Behaviors usually speak louder than words, and it takes only one nasty incident for physician–administrator relationship gains to collapse.

A number of behavioral strategies are useful in maintaining the balance between separateness and togetherness (Fiol, Pratt, and O'Connor 2009). First, it is important to encourage people to regularly express their distinctive views in public and supportive contexts. By voicing differences, people express their distinctive uniqueness; by feeling supported in voicing those differences, people experience a sense of belonging to the larger system. Second, leaders must continue to positively accentuate the differences between the groups and especially how their unique contributions make the success of the whole possible. Behaviors that make everyone feel like "we're in this together" should not be the only behaviors that are encouraged and rewarded. Rewards should also encourage behaviors that support achieving physician and administrator groups' distinctive contributions to the overarching purpose. Establishing clear objectives, observable measures, and performance-based rewards tied to the desired outcomes (e.g., clinical indicators, financial metrics, satisfaction, community reputation) is essential for motivating such behaviors.

Soften the Boundaries Between the Groups

Much of the emphasis of the PAR Process is on separating and strengthening the groups before uniting them around a common purpose. A potential criticism of this approach is that preserving and reinforcing the boundaries around each group may promote separatism and divisiveness. But evidence indicates that only when people feel secure can they feel generous or tolerant toward different others. As yet another example, studies have shown that the economic and cultural security of French and Greek Canadians is positively correlated with their view of ethnic "others" (Berry, Kalin, and Taylor 1977; Lambert, Mermigis, and Taylor 1986).

At the same time, a balance must be maintained between protecting people's need for distinctiveness and ensuring that this separateness does not evolve into ethnocentrism or an overly rigid policing of the boundaries between the groups. On August 20, 2007, Ronald Davis, then president of the most powerful and primary physician organization in the United States, the American Medical Association, reminded all physicians of their oath to "work to preserve and protect the primacy of the patient–physician relationship, and the freedom of physicians to practice medicine without undue impediment." This reflected a subtle but important change from the original statement of the oath, which was to "champion the cause of freedom in medical practice." The president noted that the words "without undue impediment" acknowledge that some autonomy is appropriately sacrificed for the sake of accountability, but the word "undue" stresses that accountability measures must be reasonable (Davis 2007). The softening of the boundaries reflected in the original oath, which had dictated complete freedom of medical practice, decreases the likelihood that the separateness of physicians would be an obstacle to needed togetherness.

A similar softening of the boundaries between the groups is reflected by hospital boards increasingly inviting physicians to be trustees and to participate in hospital decision making. The results are promising. Evidence indicates that operating margins are significantly higher for hospitals with physicians on their governing boards (Goldstein and Ward 2004). This suggests that separateness is not unduly compromised, and it makes room for simultaneous togetherness to take place.

Support Creative Abrasion

Finally, separate togetherness entails learning to deal effectively with ongoing differences and to draw from them rather than attempting to ignore or suppress them. We know that the potential for innovation and the potential for conflict both rise when people from diverse specializations interact. And we know that the healthcare world is becoming more specialized. Gerald Hirshberg, founding director of Nissan Design America, coined the term "creative abrasion" to describe how he paired designers with different priorities and work styles on a project (Hagel and Brown 2005). The clash made creative sparks fly, but it gave the different designers the freedom to let loose, knowing that the other would provide balance. What if the inevitable clashes between administrators and physicians were seen by both parties as providing balance rather than as game-stoppers?

Innovation results not from seamless interactions between highly specialized groups, but rather from challenging, stimulating, and catalytic activity where the groups meet. Interactions at the seams allow members of each group to sharpen their focus on their unique abilities; they amplify the value that each party brings to the process. At Johnson & Johnson (J&J), for example, conflict is considered a positive aspect of cross-unit collaboration (Weiss and Hughes 2005). The company has developed a council made up of representatives from the company's various units, which meets regularly to discuss differences of opinion and their strategic implications. As a result, the learning from these differences is quickly disseminated throughout J&J.

Of course, creative abrasion does not happen naturally, especially when there is a long history of distrust among the parties. When misunderstandings arise, it is easy for participants to fall back into old patterns of behavior, and the misunderstandings may harden into the old fundamental distrust. The following are a number of suggestions for preventing this from happening (Hagel and Brown 2005):

- Give each group just a few aggressive performance targets with few constraints on how the targets should be achieved.
- Address and resolve disagreements when they materialize. Do not allow them to simmer.
- Rely on forward-looking incentives rather than on backward-looking assessments.
- Define trust narrowly, focusing on the delivery of specific outcomes.
- Provide early warnings of potential performance (trust) issues, reducing the perceived risk of trusting in the first place.

- Disseminate learning from the first attempts to do this within and across units.

As another example of managing creative abrasion, Blue Cross and Blue Shield has developed a process for resolving cross-unit conflicts among managers with different perspectives and priorities (Weiss and Hughes 2005). Perspectives often clash over whether to build new capabilities, acquire them, or gain access to them through an alliance. The company uses a poster with grids, on which the managers check various boxes to indicate how they assess a particular option against a number of criteria. The format makes the criteria and trade-offs easy to compare, and the discussion that follows allows participants to see that differences in perspective often arise from access to different data or from differences in prioritization.

In sum, separate togetherness is possible, but it is wrong to assume that it will simply happen, or that once it has developed, it will maintain itself over time with no further interventions. Once you have strengthened the separate groups and brought them together in a way that draws on their unique and distinct contributions, you must maintain the balance between separateness and togetherness.

The changes in perceptions that result from the interventions we have described cannot be sustained over time without consistent and repeated attention. This is really no different than any deep change effort. To illustrate, 172 Jewish Israeli and Palestinian young people participated in a three-day intensive encounter group with the goal of easing tensions between the groups by forming interpersonal ties and learning more about one another (Bar-Natan 2005). Measures taken at the end of the three days showed that positive changes had occurred in terms of accepting the other side's narrative as legitimate and a more general acceptance of the other side. But when the same measures were taken six months later, all the positive changes had disappeared. Another study reached a similar conclusion regarding Northern Ireland's curricula of mutual understanding (Kilpatrick and Leitch 2004): Continuous intervention and ongoing reinforcement of the changes were required, especially given that those changes were under constant threat of being nullified by ongoing tensions and opposition. Shot-in-the-arm interventions will not work. Repeated reinforcement of the principles of each of the four phases is necessary to maintain separate togetherness.

WHY IT IS LIKELY TO BE RESISTED

Given the history of win-lose thinking in healthcare, it may seem completely unthinkable (even heretical) that you can work together with the "other" and still remain a separate group. And cynicism is rampant in healthcare organizations for good reasons. Attempting to forge alignment with a common overarching purpose (even among separate and secure groups) is likely to bring back memories of past integration attempts and their general failure to bring about desired results.

In many cases, old power struggles will reemerge, sometimes triggered by battles that continue beyond the boundaries of your own organization. For example, in June 2008, *Modern Healthcare* reported that a fight for authority between physicians and hospital groups about a Joint Commission standard escalated over nearly five years (DerGurahian 2008). The standard outlined the fundamental relationship between hospital administration and medical staff. Doctors felt the standard denied them self-governance, and that medical staffs would not have the independent voice they need to speak directly to the board when they saw room for improvement. Such extended public battles can suck people back into old patterns of thinking and behaving, making it difficult, if not impossible, for them to envision collaborating.

A final reason physicians and administrators may resist engaging in the process of developing separate togetherness is their perception that the common purpose, which is meant to draw them together, is not common at all, but rather reflects the interests of the other group. Even when the overarching purpose truly represents the interests of all involved, people will often perceive the current reality through historical lenses, which may distort their perception and block their engagement.

HOW TO MOVE THROUGH THE RESISTANCE

There are a number of ways to move people through their resistance to engaging in separate togetherness. Naturally, people will need regular reassurance that their separate autonomy is not lost. They also need reminders of their dependence on one another. Beyond these reminders, we offer specific suggestions for moving through resistance.

Reinforce the Encompassing Nature of Your Statement of Purpose

At the top of our list of recommendations is constant reinforcement of the encompassing nature of the common purpose. The eventual statement of purpose cannot be seen as competing with the interests of either group, and it cannot be seen as belonging to either group alone. If the statement of purpose is perceived as a threat to the interests and values of one group, the threatened individuals will resist letting go of their past understanding of who they are, who the "other" is, and how they should relate, blocking any possibility of a new way of interacting. For example, if bottom-line margin is perceived to be the centerpiece of the overarching purpose, one would expect clinical team members to resist. Similarly, a person in finance is not likely to support a purpose he or she perceives as focused on providing the best clinical care at any cost.

Establish Clear Sponsorship in Each Group

Sponsors are leaders who legitimize change in organizations through words, behaviors, and deployment of resources. It is important that sponsors demonstrate their support for the new compacts and for simultaneous group separateness and togetherness in private and public conversations. Members of the board, physician, and administrative transition teams are likely group sponsors early on, but others may emerge over time.

As we have noted, credibility is the most important criterion for a group's sponsor to effectively reduce resistance, and credibility is enhanced when the sponsor is considered "one of us." The president of Cedars-Sinai Medical Center once sought a way to increase physician hand-washing compliance to 90 percent, as mandated by The Joint Commisssion. Catching people washing their hands and giving them a $10 Starbucks card increased compliance from 65 percent to 80 percent. At a Chief of Staff Advisory Committee meeting, one of the epidemiologists gave physicians agar plates, cultured their hands, and photographed the images. A photograph with many colonies of bacteria was made into a screen saver for every computer in the hospital. Hand-washing compliance shot up to nearly 100 percent, where it remained some years later (Dubner and Levitt 2006). Each of your groups needs credible sponsorship to applaud people who behave according to the principles of separate togetherness and to provide leadership when resistance arises.

Finally, if resistance continues during this final phase of the PAR Process, more work may be needed on prior phases to gain readiness, to disentangle the negative connections between the groups, or to develop each group's sense of security in its own unique distinctiveness. Remember, the conditions of each phase are critical to the success of the subsequent one.

DISSEMINATION OF SEPARATE TOGETHERNESS BEYOND OPINION LEADERS

At first blush, the principles of separate togetherness seem completely paradoxical. It is only after observing that those principles can be implemented and maintained that the majority will likely wish to participate. Once again, we recommend that you begin the process by drawing on the opinion leaders from each of your three transition teams (physician, administrator, and board). If the members of the transition teams model the principles of (1) respecting the differences between the groups, (2) recognizing the value of combining the differences, (3) identifying a creative but realistic purpose, and (4) preserving the identity of the groups in the process, others in the organization are more likely to follow.

CHAPTER SUMMARY

This chapter described the fourth and final phase of the PAR Process, which focuses on aligning physicians and administrators (with the support of the board) around a joint purpose while promoting their security in the separateness and distinctiveness of their own groups. We clarified why neither *togetherness* alone nor *separateness* alone will lead to success—both are needed simultaneously. The chapter discussed what separate togetherness entails and emphasized the importance of establishing an ongoing process of reinforcing the principles of each of the four phases in order to sustain it. The assessment exercises at the end of this chapter will give you a sense of the extent to which you have achieved separate togetherness at your organization, and the exercises for promoting separate togetherness summarize the steps for achieving this outcome.

Separate Togetherness at Louis Martin Community Hospital
The three transition teams at LMCH met to develop the first draft of a system-wide purpose statement that would encompass the interests of each group. After numerous iterations and a great deal of feedback from their peers, they developed the following statement: "Best place to give and get

---

(Continued on following page)

care, now and in the future." The trustees, administrators, and physicians at LMCH all bought into this statement of purpose, made it their own, and were able to see how it required each of their group's unique contributions.

To ensure that people would continue to adhere to the principles of separate togetherness, a team (consisting of members from each of the three groups) was formed with the charge of articulating a new compact between physicians and administrators. The new compact reflected the principles of separate togetherness (respect the differences, recognize the value from combining the differences, identify a creative but realistic purpose, and preserve the identity of the groups as they align around that purpose). It included details about new ways of thinking, speaking, and behaving with one another. It identified areas where prior rigid boundaries between the groups needed to be relaxed to accommodate the new coequal partnership, and it established time lines and processes for ensuring accountability.

All of this was accomplished with the support of most of the trustees, administrators, and physicians. A few administrators and physicians who were not able to adjust to the new compact chose to leave. Overall, the leadership at LMCH was thrilled. By fostering strong and qualified leadership in each group, senior management, physician leaders, and trustees could begin to make tough decisions as equal partners. Resource allocation was no longer based on who could shout the loudest, but on formally constructed business plans developed by the partners.

The biggest struggle for leaders at LMCH has been to treat the inevitable clashes that still arise between physicians and administrators as creative abrasion. When conflicts surface, the knee-jerk reaction still seems to be that somehow the process has failed. To address this challenge, they have developed a learning council with representation from the three groups, charged with monitoring relations and turning conflictive situations into learning opportunities.

The results have been dramatic, and 2008 was a turning point. Financial stability improved, total physician compensation increased as physician productivity increased, physician satisfaction improved as their suggestions for clinical improvements were acted on, and employee satisfaction scores went up as workplace tensions dissipated, turnover decreased, and patient satisfaction spiraled upward.

SELF-ASSESSMENT EXERCISES

Assessing Separate Togetherness at Your Organization

Please respond to each statement in Sections 1, 2, and 3 by indicating your level of agreement on a scale ranging from Strongly Disagree (1) to Strongly Agree (5).

Depending on who is completing the assessment, Section 1 will provide information about trustees' opinions regarding how well they are following the principles of separate togetherness, *or* administrators' and physicians' opinions regarding how well trustees are following those principles. Similarly, Section 2 will provide information about physicians' opinions regarding how well they are following the principles of separate togetherness, *or* administrators' and trustees' opinions regarding how well physicians are following the principles. And finally, Section 3 will provide information about administrators' opinions regarding how well they are following the principles of separate togetherness, *or* physicians' and trustees' opinions regarding how well administrators are following the principles.

Section 1: Board members

Board members demonstrate ongoing commitment to the integrative purpose of the health system. _____

Board members consistently emphasize differences in the value contributed by physicians and administrators in positive ways. _____

Board members regularly support physicians and administrators in making decisions in areas in which they have the greatest level of expertise. _____

Board members demonstrate ongoing commitment to the long-term well-being of the medical staff, the administrative team, and the organization as a whole. _____

Board members demonstrate ongoing commitment to exceptional clinical and financial outcomes.   _____

Board members are very proud to be members of the board and equally proud to be associated with physicians and administrators at this hospital.   _____

Average score for Section 1   _____

Section 2: Physicians

Physicians demonstrate ongoing commitment to the integrative purpose of the health system.   _____

Physicians consistently emphasize differences in the value contributed by physicians and administrators in positive ways.   _____

Physicians regularly support both groups in making decisions in areas in which they have the greatest level of expertise.   _____

Physicians demonstrate ongoing commitment to the long-term well-being of the medical staff and of the organization as a whole.   _____

Physicians demonstrate ongoing commitment to exceptional financial and clinical outcomes.   _____

Physicians are very proud to be members of the medical staff and equally proud to be associated with this hospital.   _____

Average score for Section 2   _____

Section 3: Administrators

Administrators demonstrate ongoing commitment to
the integrative purpose of the health system.   _____

Administrators consistently emphasize differences in
the value contributed by physicians and administrators in positive ways.   _____

Administrators regularly support both groups in
making decisions in areas in which they have the
greatest level of expertise.   _____

Administrators demonstrate ongoing commitment to
the long-term well-being of the members of the
administrative team and of the organization as a
whole.   _____

Administrators demonstrate ongoing commitment to
exceptional clinical and financial outcomes.   _____

Administrators are very proud to be members of the
administrative team and equally proud to be associated with this hospital.   _____

Average score for Section 3   _____

Please average the scores for Sections 1, 2, and 3 separately.

The average score of Section 1 reveals how well trustees believe
their group is following the principles of separate togetherness, *or*
administrators' or physicians' opinions regarding how trustees are
following those principles.

The average score of Section 2 reveals how well physicians believe
their group is following the principles of separate togetherness, *or*

administrators' or trustees' opinions regarding how well physicians are following those principles.

The average score of Section 3 reveals how well administrators believe their group is following the principles of separate togetherness, *or* physicians' or trustees' opinions regarding how well administrators are following those principles.

How does your organization look when evaluated against these statements? High average scores indicate that your organization may have done the work required to progress toward separate togetherness, where both physicians and administrators are committed to their own group's success and the success of the entire organization. However, any average score lower than four (4) suggests the need for serious consideration, if not action to further develop separate togetherness. What changes would be helpful as you move toward developing separate togetherness?

———————————————————————————

———————————————————————————

———————————————————————————

———————————————————————————

———————————————————————————

———————————————————————————

EXERCISES FOR PROMOTING SEPARATE TOGETHERNESS

If people are highly resistant to the promotion of separate togetherness, please begin with the following steps:

1. Reinforce the encompassing nature of the overarching purpose that is being identified for the organization, with continual reminders that each group's interests will be represented.

2. Emphasize the different roles that physicians and administrators carry out at your hospital, and connect the dots for them by demonstrating how those roles interact and support each other as they align with the larger purpose.

3. Ensure that sponsors for each group reward those who follow the principles of separate togetherness, and model the principles to those who are still resistant to new patterns of thinking, speaking, and behaving.

As resistance lessens and awareness of the benefits of separate togetherness increases, begin the following exercises to further promote it.

4. Articulate an overarching purpose for your hospital/health system that requires each group's distinctive contributions. A purpose provides a common cause with which the system is aligned, rather than a goal that can be achieved. The following is an example of a unifying purpose statement: "Best place to give and get care, now and in the future."

Follow the principles of separate togetherness in developing your statement of purpose.

- Respect the differences.

- Recognize the value from combining the differences.

- Be creative but realistic.

- Preserve the identity of the groups.

Emphasize publicly each group's contribution to the common purpose.

Align all strategic initiatives with the common purpose.

Refer often to the purpose when explaining leadership strategies.

Determine the mechanisms required to coordinate the distinctive and separate contributions of each group. For examples of integrating mechanisms, please refer to the material presented earlier in this chapter.

5. Rewrite the old compacts.

What have been the spoken or unspoken assumptions about what physicians at your organization give? What do they get? What have been the spoken or unspoken assumptions about what administrators at your organization give? What do they get?

Consider what parts of those old compacts are becoming obsolete. Why?

How do these compacts affect the health system's ability to respond to market forces? How do they affect each group's ability to contribute to effective responses?

Following the four principles of separate togetherness, rewrite the compacts between physicians and administrators at your hospital.

Create a form that lists the four principles of separate togetherness on the left side, and then lists each group's gives and gets, taking into account each of the principles. An example of the outline of a compact clarifying what physicians give and get is shown in Table 8.2.

The new compacts will have little effect unless organizational systems are put in place to ensure implementation and ongoing monitoring, using the following steps:

- Develop new or refine existing policies to be consistent with the new compacts.

- Ensure that resource allocations are aligned with the new compacts.

- Establish measurement and feedback systems to monitor the extent to which each group is living up to the new compacts.

Table 8.2 Sample Compact Outline Showing What Physicians Give and Get

Principles	Give	Get
Respect the differences	Clinical priorities that respect administrative interests	Managerial guidelines that respect the right of physicians to make care decisions
Acknowledge value from combining	Constructive physician input into hospital planning	Greater voice in the future of the hospital
Identify a creative but realistic purpose	Commitment to championing excellent patient care without undue impediments	Administrative support for delivering excellent care without undue impediments
Preserve group identity	Value the expertise of the administrative team	Be valued as medical experts

- Tie some part of the compensation and reward system to meeting the expectations of the new compacts.

6. Foster new ways of thinking and speaking.

This begins with physician and administrative leaders and trustees systematically modeling effective language by using referents to highlight the different group memberships.

- Link self and others by clarifying what "we" share in common. "We" are
  - providing extraordinary care
  - improving patient safety
  - committed to long-term community healthcare

- Unite against common threats/enemies. "We" must battle together against
  - government regulators
  - greedy payers
  - misguided community leaders

- Separate self from others by clarifying differences between the groups: "We" provide excellent clinical care and "they" ensure financial viability.

7. Foster new ways of behaving.

This begins with leaders

- encouraging people to publicly, responsibly, and respectfully express their differences and supporting them in doing so;

- continuing to accentuate differences between physicians and administrators in positive ways;

- establishing objectives for each group and for the larger unit; and

- measuring and rewarding unique and distinctive contributions to the whole.

8. Soften the boundaries between the groups.

Invite groups of physicians, administrators, and trustees to meet separately to discuss which aspects of each group's autonomy or separateness may impinge on the success of the larger unit. Develop a list of three to five substantive areas in which your group is willing to soften the boundaries and give up some of its autonomy to more fully contribute to the larger purpose.

Examples of boundary softening include

- inviting increasing number of physicians to be trustees,

- inviting trustees and administrators to attend medical executive committee meetings, and

- encouraging joint strategic planning and shared hospital decision making.

Transition teams should then meet and exchange offers of ways to soften the boundaries between them.

A team made up of representatives of each group can then develop a specific plan for implementing the agreed-to changes.

9. Support creative abrasion.

Invite groups of physicians and administrators to each develop a few aggressive performance targets with few constraints on how the targets should be achieved.

Clarify processes for addressing and resolving disagreements when they materialize.

Rely on forward-looking incentives related to aligning around the common purpose, rather than on backward-looking assessments.

Define trust narrowly, focusing on its implications for the delivery of specific outcomes under specific conditions.

Provide early warnings of potential performance (trust) issues, reducing the perceived risks of trusting in the first place.

Disseminate the learning from this process within and across peer groups.

PART III

WHERE TO BEGIN, AND HOW TO SUSTAIN THE SUCCESSES

CHAPTER 9

Ten Steps to Healthy Hospital–Physician Relations

Face reality as it is, not as it was or as you wish it to be.

—Jack Welch,
Former Chairman/CEO, General Electric

Now this is not the end. It is not even the beginning of the end. But it is, perhaps, the end of the beginning.

—Sir Winston Churchill,
Former Prime Minister, United Kingdom

It can't be this hard, and I don't want it to take this long. Certainly it must be simpler to entice physicians and administrators to work together effectively. After all, as the argument goes, they take care of the same patients and serve the same communities. We just need to try one more visioning retreat with a better facilitator this year, or to try out that new structural form described in this year's healthcare bestseller.

SO GOES THE LOGIC of those who have not yet given up on the traditional solutions to building physician–administrator partnerships. The upside of these old approaches is that they can be implemented far more rapidly than the PAR Process we have described. In addition, it is easy to rationalize going down these paths, because they are crowded with other healthcare leaders who are also pursuing quick fixes to their long-term problems. However, just as short-term diets and exercise programs do not provide solutions for long-term abuse of our bodies, long-term tensions in physician–hospital relations are likely to require long-term, ongoing investments in the healing process. As we reviewed in chapters 2 and 3, the traditional structural and visioning approaches for building hospital–physician relations have typically been found wanting. Consistent with the quote from Welch that begins this chapter, it may be more productive to face reality as it is than as it was or as you wish it to be.

By the time John Gray's book *Men Are from Mars, Women Are from Venus* appeared in paperback, more than 14 million of us had purchased the book to better understand how our partners differed from us and how that understanding could help us build lasting, committed relationships. Weary of the approach presented in thousands of books touting the similarities between the sexes, people were eager for Gray's message, which emphasized our differences and how to capitalize on them.

The message of our book is built on a similar premise, but the analogy is not perfect. Understanding how your partner differs from you is straightforward compared with the challenges of understanding how physicians differ from hospital administrators and how those differences can be used to create advantages. Physicians understand themselves to be many different things, as do administrators, and members of each group often do not cohere around a common identity until they are faced with a threat from the "other." The PAR Process first creates readiness to untangle the negative connections, then unites and strengthens each group. Only after these steps have been accomplished does it address the question of how the separate groups can coordinate to, together, bring about desired results.

Although the four phases of the PAR Process can move your physician and administrative groups from negative entanglement to sustained collaboration, the steps require pre- and post-process support (see boxes). Before you engage your people in a PAR Process, four pre-process steps must be taken. Only then are the four phases of the PAR Process likely to be successful. And when the four phases have been completed, a number of post-process steps are required to ensure sustained success.

Steps for Support Throughout the PAR Process

Pre–PAR Process Support

Step 1   Obtain senior sponsorship.

Step 2   Engage neutral buffers in the form of a third party to facilitate moving beyond distrust.

Step 3   Present a map of the entire PAR process to physicians, administrators, and trustees.

Step 4   Identify transition teams.

PAR Process

Step 5   Develop physician, administrator, and trustee readiness to begin.

Step 6   Disentangle the negative connections between physicians and administrators.

Step 7   Strengthen each group's security about its own distinctive value.

Step 8   Promote separate togetherness.

(Continued on following page)

(Continued from previous page)

Post–PAR Process Support

Step 9   Ensure that ongoing strategies for physician–administrator integration adhere to principles of separate togetherness.

Step 10 Maintain vigilance in order to sustain the successes.

PRE–PAR PROCESS SUPPORT

Step 1: Senior Sponsorship

Sponsors are individuals with formal or informal authority who legitimize new ways of thinking and behaving (O'Connor and Fiol 2006). These individuals have the power to make what they say stick. For example, either the hospital board or the CEO may establish sponsorship by controlling the resources needed to pay for the processes required to alter the way physicians and administrators relate to each other. Physicians who have high credibility among their peers due to their informal leadership or clinical skills may similarly establish sponsorship simply by offering their opinions.

PAR Process success depends on strong sponsorship from physicians, administrators, and board members. Leaders from any of these groups can block the process. While outsiders may play a useful facilitating role, internal sponsorship is critical to success.

How does one develop and maintain this support? Although one may simply ask for it, asking alone is unlikely to succeed in sustaining required sponsorship throughout the PAR Process. A more effective strategy involves identifying the outcomes to which specific physician, administrator, and trustee sponsors are committed (e.g., medical or financial excellence) and then explaining or demonstrating how improved collaboration will provide a pathway to those outcomes.

The exercises presented in Chapter 5 are valuable in developing and expanding support for the PAR Process, but gaining the legitimacy needed to engage in those activities requires up-front sponsorship in each of the critical groups. Investments in assessing, expanding, and sustaining that sponsorship are essential to the long-term success of the PAR Process.

Step 2: Neutral Buffers

Roughly half of all managers do not trust their leaders, and more than four out of five Americans have only some confidence in the people running major corporations (Hurley 2006). The situation may be even worse in healthcare, where physicians and administrators often operate from very different assumptions. For example, physicians often see administrators as isolated from the real pressures of patient care, paid for nonproductive work (e.g., meetings), and always worried about costs; and administrators report that physicians lack a big-picture mind-set, are unwilling to make time for administrative tasks but do not trust others to do them, have a hard time making group decisions (e.g., lack leadership), and function as if other healthcare workers are less valuable (Weber 2006). Building on these differences, each group may easily fall into unconsciously operating as if "we are right and they are wrong" and "if something goes wrong, it must be their fault."

When this occurs, listening to members of the other group carefully with a sincere desire to understand their views becomes challenging. Behaviors of the "other" are often misinterpreted based on preconceptions, and old patterns of distrust are used as filters in making sense of their actions. For example, if I already believe that the CEO cannot be trusted, I may reject new, even well-intentioned, offers, believing that there must be a catch.

Under these conditions, even those physician and administrative leaders with the best intentions have difficulty disentangling the negative connections between the groups, since information exchange is frequently interpreted through old perspectives. As we noted earlier, PAR Process success depends heavily on sponsorship from both groups. If leaders from either group block the process, neutral outsiders may convince these groups to consider new alternatives and to move beyond their well-entrenched perspectives. This is especially true during the early phases of the process (readiness, disentangling, and security development) when relationships are strained, distrust is still high, and group-level security is still limited.

Step 3: Map of the Process

Having driven less than one mile of our 900-plus-mile trip from Boston, Massachusetts, to Chattanooga, Tennessee, it was discouraging to hear our two-and-a-half-year-old son ask, "Are we there yet?" Many of us have had similar experiences in traveling with young children who possess a limited understanding of time and distance. Similar challenges arise with physicians and administrators if the PAR Process is not clearly understood before beginning the intervention. When leaders are under the illusion that the process will rapidly take them to what they really want to do (e.g., rewrite physician–hospital compacts, partner in strategic thinking), participants become discouraged by the time, commitment, and resources required. Clearly mapping out the phases of the process, explaining the actions it will take to complete those phases, and building realistic expectations for how long it will take to heal relationships that have long been strained are essential to maintaining the commitment required for success.

In addition to discouraging false starts from those who are not yet ready to make the investments the PAR Process requires, mapping out the phases physicians and administrators will pass through can be encouraging to those who are ready to make the journey. Without clarity about what the foundational phases will lead to, it is unlikely that physicians and administrators who are locked in battle will even begin to relinquish their positions. Only when leaders are clear about the ultimate payoffs will the steps along the way seem worth the time and energy.

Step 4: Transition Teams

As we have repeatedly noted throughout this book, not everyone is ready to adopt new ideas and behaviors at the same time or on the same schedule. As with any innovation, the PAR Process can be expected to spread among innovators, opinion leaders, early majority, late majority, and traditionalists in a progressive and expanding sequence over time (Rogers 2003). Physician, administrator, and board transition teams are essential to facilitating this diffusion. These teams should be formed early in Phase One and should play an active role in spreading ideas throughout the healthcare system.

The three to seven members of each transition team should be chosen by their peers based on (1) possessing a high level of credibility with those peers and (2) being relatively open-minded and able to embrace new ways of thinking and behaving. Members of the physician transition team should be the first physicians to go through each of the phases of the PAR Process and should lead the dissemination of what they have learned at each phase to other physicians in the system. Similarly, members of the administrator transition team should be the first administrators to go through each phase and should lead the dissemination of what they have learned. In addition to these responsibilities with their peers, the board transition team should provide oversight of the PAR Process, ensuring ongoing senior sponsorship.

PAR PROCESS

Each phase of the PAR Process is a building block for those that follow. As noted in earlier chapters, successfully moving forward requires

1. readiness to begin,
2. disentangled negative connections,
3. separate group security, and
4. separate togetherness that makes collaboration possible.

All healthcare systems may not need to start the PAR Process at the beginning. For example, they may not need to develop readiness if it already exists. Similarly, disentangling negative connections may not be necessary if current physician–administrator relationships are respectful. It is essential, however, to know whether each of these conditions exists before skipping any of the phases. The assessment exercises provided in chapters 5 through 8 allow you to clarify where your organization is starting from and what actions it should initially take to move forward.

Although we have presented the four phases of the PAR Process as if they were linear, with each phase being completed before beginning the one that follows, the phases typically overlap one another. For example, successfully disentangling negative connections (Phase Two) requires that physicians and administrators give up the negative security they derive from knowing that they are right because the other group is wrong. Beginning the third phase of developing separate group security within each group based on its distinctive positive contributions can therefore encourage people to completely disentangle by letting go of their negative sources of security.

The phases also overlap in that different physicians and different administrators will be experiencing different phases at the same time. As noted above, transition team members are responsible for beginning each phase and then diffusing the resulting ideas and behaviors throughout their early majority, late majority, and traditionalist peers.

Step 5: Readiness to Begin

Readiness for the PAR Process implies a high level of commitment to de-escalating conflict. It involves a steadfast dedication to significantly improving physician–hospital relations. While it does not mean that people want to give up old ways of thinking and behaving, it does mean that they are willing to change because they are unwilling or unable to bear the ongoing battles, or because they see the possibilities of a new way of relating to each other.

The readiness phase of the PAR Process moves people past the intractable righteousness that easily paralyzes physician–hospital relations and begins to develop in people the dedication required to de-escalate costly conflicts. Successfully moving through this phase requires physicians and administrators to see a threat to things they value if they do not give up their old ways of relating, great benefits as a result of doing so, and lowered risks involved in trying new ways of interacting with each other.

Step 6: Disentangled Negative Connections

The purpose of the second phase of the PAR Process is to disentangle the negative connections between physicians and administrators by breaking down the stereotypes that lock them into zero-sum perspectives. Disentangling requires temporarily suspending old beliefs (e.g., when something goes wrong, it must be their fault) and a growing reluctance to overly simplify reality (e.g., we are always right and they are always wrong).

If readiness to begin (the result of the prior phase) is not present, attempts to disentangle the negative connections between physicians and administrators are likely to seem too inconsistent with historical ways of thinking about each other, to appear to be not worth the risk/costs, and to be resisted. To increase the chances that group members will shift their attention from their negative views of each other to a more productive focus on their own group's distinctive value, we described a number of helpful steps during the disentangling phase, including (1) transferring learning from similar conflicts in other industries, (2) identifying common ground between physicians and administrators, and (3) generating small win projects that demonstrate the capacity of the groups to work together effectively.

Step 7: Separate Group Security

Members of physician and administrative groups often lack a sense of security about their collective value as a group. This insecurity results from fragmentation in departments and competition among specialties and subspecialties. The purpose of the separate group security phase of the PAR Process is to develop satisfaction, pride, and a sense of belonging within each of these groups. The objective is for physicians and administrators to feel secure about their group's distinctive value and unique contribution to the healthcare system. Security requires moving beyond negative comparisons (e.g., we're good because we're not like "them") to a focus on positive contribution (e.g., we're good because of our distinctive, valuable contributions).

To the degree that each group feels secure in its own distinctive value, physicians and administrators will feel less threatened by the strength and success of the other group, and the possibility for each to focus on their respective clinical and administrative dreams will increase. We described a number of steps that will increase the chances that physicians and administrators will come together around their own group's distinctive contributions, including (1) formally articulating the priorities of each group, (2) regularly publicizing their distinctive contributions, and (3) developing clear measures to document the value each group provides.

Step 8: Separate Togetherness

The purpose of the separate togetherness phase of the PAR Process is to align secure physician and secure administrative groups around a unifying purpose, while maintaining the strength and security of each group. Separate togetherness requires that members of each group see themselves as distinct and separate from the "other" while collaborating with the "other" toward a common purpose. When disentangling and separate group security (the prior two phases of the PAR Process) have not been accomplished, promoting togetherness alone is likely to lead to resistance since physicians and administrators may not view themselves as "all in this together." Similarly, promoting separateness alone is likely to lead to failure since the combined expertise of secure physicians and secure administrators is essential to sustained success.

When separate group security is not present, supporting separate togetherness typically appears too threatening and seems not worth the risk. As a result, it will be resisted. Helpful steps for promoting separate togetherness include (1) articulating an overarching purpose for the system as a whole, (2) fostering new ways of communicating, and (3) rewriting old hospital–physician compacts.

The foundation built by successful completion of the four phases of the PAR Process opens the door to a major competitive advantage: powerful and distinctively different healthcare groups within your system working together to address today's ever-changing healthcare challenges. At best, however, the relationship successes you achieve through implementation of the PAR Process may simply provide, in Churchill's words, the "end of the beginning." Consistent with the second law of thermodynamics, without ongoing investments, disorder in a system tends to increase over time. In the best relationships, transgressions will be perceived, and ongoing work is required if stability is to be maintained and expansion is to occur. Post–PAR Process support is needed to sustain the gains the PAR Process has achieved.

POST–PAR PROCESS SUPPORT

Step 9: Ensure That Ongoing Strategies Adhere to Principles of Separate Togetherness

As we stated in Chapter 4, the completion of the PAR Process phases provides the foundation for successful application of traditional integration approaches. For example, although transparent information sharing by physicians and administrators has often been recommended, the vulnerability required for its success is seldom present in negatively entangled groups that are locked in intractable conflict. This strategy is more likely to succeed, however, if the negative connections between the groups have been disentangled and if each group feels secure in its own distinctive value. Similarly, shared decision making seems unlikely to be productive unless both groups are secure in their separate strengths and the togetherness resulting from parallel commitments to the health system's well-being.

Any of the failed structural and visioning integrative approaches that we reviewed in chapters 2 and 3 are much more likely to succeed once separate togetherness has been achieved. Although each of these traditional approaches has suffered its share of humiliating failures in the healthcare field, each can be used to build toward sustained success if the proper foundation has been laid. That foundation consists of secure and separate groups of physicians and administrators who are ready to move along parallel paths toward creating a common dream.

The structural form (e.g., joint venture, salaried physicians) of separate togetherness is less important than adherence to its principles. Clear answers to the question of which structural arrangements are best do not seem to exist. For example, one study reported that 30 percent of New England hospitals are working on at least one joint venture with physicians, but only 35 percent of those involved in a joint venture say that it succeeds in aligning physicians and hospitals (Haugh 2005). And while hospitals around the country generally attempted to rid themselves of physician practices because they tended to be losing propositions, North Carolina–based Novant Health saw its large physician practice (Forsyth Medical Group) move from red to black ink after it turned to its physicians for leadership. Dr. Jack Thomas, one of the employed physicians, stated that "it doesn't feel like we're employed. It feels like we're running a practice with a great deal of support" (Norbut 2003). That is the key: People must feel that their uniqueness is maintained and their distinct contributions are supported, while collaborating toward a common vision with the "other."

Step 10: Vigilance

We have delineated an uncommon path away from the dysfunctional and destructive relations that often characterize physician and administrator interactions and toward collaboration of the distinct and separate groups. Managing the polarities of such an apparent paradox as separate togetherness is never-ending work. Backsliding into old ways of thinking and behaving is always a danger, which makes ongoing vigilance and corrective actions necessary. So do not enter into this process believing it will be an easy fix to the challenges you face in managing your physician–hospital relations. To manage such polarities, you need patience and a high tolerance for ambiguity. Are you able to accept that the job of managing the delicate balance between separateness and togetherness is never done? And are you and your people prepared to really believe in and publicly communicate that there is no single answer to the question of "who we are" as a health provider system?

Historically, administrators and clinicians have battled over which group should be the captain of the ship (Romano 2004b). We have turned that age-old argument on its head. For relations between administrators and hospitals to be successful and sustainable, each side must captain its own ship, and the ships must be moving in a common direction. Despite solid evidence from numerous arenas that supports our argument, it is not immediately intuitive. To align both groups around a common purpose, you must first disentangle the negative connections between them and then strengthen each as a separate entity. Following a nonintuitive and nonobvious path instead of common wisdom requires creativity, insight, and courage. But since common wisdom is not bringing about the hoped-for results, it is time to look for answers in new places.

References

Abrams, L. C., R. Cross, E. Lesser, and D. Z. Levin. 2003. "Nurturing Interpersonal Trust in Knowledge-Sharing Networks." *Academy of Management Executive* 17 (4): 64–77.

Ackermann, M. 2006. "Health Care Big Retirement Fear, Poll." *American Banker* 171 (248): 7.

Advisory Board Company. 2007. "Hospitals Design Strategies to Head off Physician Turf Battles." [Online article; retrieved 5/30/07.] www.advisory.com/login/login.aspx?URL=/members/default.asp?contentID=66815&collectionID=4&program=1&filename=66815.xml.

———. 1999. "Physician Survey." Washington, DC: Advisory Board Company.

Algeo, D. 1997. "Doctors Hurl Gauntlet." *Denver Post*, November 10, E-01.

Anderson, R. 2003. "Building Hospital–Physician Relationships Through Servant Leadership." *Frontiers of Health Services Management* 20 (2): 43–47.

Annison, M. H., and D. S. Wilford. 1998. *Trust Matters: New Directions in Health Care Leadership.* San Francisco: Jossey-Bass.

Asch, S. M., E. A. Kerr, J. Keesey, J. L. Adams, C. M. Setodji, S. Malik, and E. A. McGlynn. 2006. "Who Is at Greatest Risk for Receiving Poor-Quality Health Care?" *The New England Journal of Medicine* 354 (11): 1147–56.

Ashforth, B. E., and F. Mael. 1989. "Social Identity Theory and the Organization." *Academy of Management Review* 14 (1): 20–39.

Atchison, T. A., and J. S. Bujak. 2001. *Leading Transformational Change: The Physician–Executive Partnership.* Chicago: Health Administration Press.

Baicker, K. 2006. "Improving Incentives in Health Care Spending." *Business Economics* 41 (2): 21–25.

Bard, M. A., M. L. Buehler, A. L. Epstein, D. B. Nash, and J. P. O'Connor. 2002. "Strong Partners Make Good Partners: Insights About Physician–Hospital Relationships from a Study of Physician Executives." *Disease Management* 5 (3): 137–42.

Bar-Natan, I. 2005. "Does Friendship Between Adversaries Generalize?" Doctoral dissertation, Haifa University.

Bazzoli, G. J., L. Dynan, L. R. Burns, and C. Yap. 2004. "Two Decades of Organizational Change in Health Care: What Have We Learned? *Medical Care Research and Review* 61 (3): 247–331.

Berry, J. W., R. Kalin, and D. M. Taylor. 1977. *Multiculturalism and Ethnic Attitudes in Canada.* Ottawa: Minister of Supply and Services.

Berwick, D. 2003. "Disseminating Innovations in Health Care." *JAMA* 289 (15): 1969–75.

Bogue, R. J., J. G. Guarneri, M. Reed, K. Bradley, and J. Hughes. 2006. "Secrets of Physician Satisfaction." *Physician Executive* 32 (6): 30–39.

Bottles, K. 2000. "Why Are Physicians So Angry?" *Physician Executive* 26 (5): 44–48.

Brett, J., K. Behfar, and M. Kern. 2006. "Managing Multicultural Teams." *Harvard Business Review* (November): 84–91.

Brett, J. M., and M. Janssens. 2006. "Cultural Intelligence in Global Teams: A Fusion Model of Collaboration." *Group and Organization Management* 31 (1): 124–53.

Broermann, R. A. 2003. "Straight Talk: New Approaches in Healthcare: The Outpatient Market: Protect Important Market Share." *Modern Healthcare* 33 (43): 29–32.

Budetti, P. P., S. M. Shortell, T. M. Waters, J. A. Alexander, L. R. Burns, R. Gillies, and H. Zuckerman. 2002. "Physician and Health System Integration: Public and Private Policies Push Physicians and Health Systems Together, But They Can Also Drive Them Apart." *Health Affairs* 21 (1): 203–10.

Bujak, J. S. 2008. *Inside the Physician Mind: Finding Common Ground with Doctors.* Chicago: Health Administration Press.

———. 2003. "How to Improve Hospital–Physician Relationships." *Frontiers of Health Services Management* 20 (2): 3–21.

Burda, D. 2008. "Special Report: Labor Intensive." *Modern Healthcare* (November 17): 26.

Cameron, K. 1997. "Techniques for Making Organizations Effective." In *Enhancing Organizational Performance,* edited by D. Druckman, J. Singer, and H. Van Cott, 39–64. Washington, DC: National Academy Press.

Carlson, J. 2009. "New Year's Stress: ACHE Survey Shows Finances Lead Execs' Concerns." *Modern Healthcare* (January 12): 14.

———. 2008. "It's All Downhill from Here." *Modern Healthcare*, (November 17): 6.

Casanova, J. 2004. "The Docs Are in Charge: Physician Executives Branch Out to Lead a Diverse Array of Institutions." [Online article; retrieved 10/5/04.] www.modernhealthcare.com/apps/pbcs.dll/article?AID=/200 30428/REG/304280317&nocache=1.

Chernow, M., R. Hirth, and D. Cutler. 2003. "Increased Spending on Health Care: How Much Can the United States Afford?" *Health Affairs* 22 (4): 15–25.

Clarke, J. R., J. C. Lerner, and W. Marella. 2007. "The Role for Leaders of Health Care Organizations in Patient Safety." *American Journal of Medical Quality* 22 (5): 311–18.

Clevenger, K. 2007. "Team Building Retreats." *Nursing Management* 38 (4): 23–24.

Clinton, W. 2008. Remarks by President Bill Clinton at Portland State University Commencement. [Online article; retrieved 4/1/08.] www.shusterman.com/prez.html.

Coddington, D. C., E. A. Fischer, K. D. Moore, and R. L. Clarke. 2000. *Beyond Managed Care: How Consumers and Technology Are Changing the Future of Healthcare.* San Francisco: Jossey-Bass.

Cohn, K. H. 2006. *Collaborate for Success: Breakthrough Strategies for Engaging Physicians, Nurses, and Hospital Executives.* Chicago: Health Administration Press.

———. 2005. *Better Communication for Better Care: Mastering Physician–Administrator Collaboration.* Chicago: Health Administration Press.

Cohn, K. H., and T. R. Allyn. 2005. "Making Hospital–Physician Collaboration Work." *HFM Magazine* 59 (10): 102–8.

Cohn, K. H., T. R. Allyn, R. H. Rosenfield, and R. Schwartz. 2005. "Overview of Physician–Hospital Ventures." *American Journal of Surgery* 189 (1): 4–10.

Cohn, K. H., S. L. Gill, and R. W. Schwartz. 2005. "Gaining Hospital Administrators' Attention: Ways to Improve Physician–Hospital Management Dialogue." *Surgery* 137 (2): 132–40.

Colias, M. 2004. "Connecting the Dots: Verispan's Annual 'IHN 100' Ranks Organizations That Are Using Higher Degrees of Integration to Excel Clinically and Financially." *Modern Healthcare* 34 (5): 25–29.

Collins, J. C., and J. I. Porras. 1994. *Built to Last: Successful Habits of Visionary Companies.* New York: Harper Business.

Colliver, V. 2005. "Excessive Medical Expenses: Study Finds that Half of Health Care Dollars Are Wasted." *San Francisco Chronicle*, February 9. [Online article; retrieved 2/9/05.] http://www.sfgate.com/cgi-bin/article.cgi?f= /c/a/2005/02/09/BUG7RB7VEM1.DTL&hw=Excessive+Me dical+Expenses+Study+Finds+that+Half+of+Health+Care+D ollars+are+Wasted&sn=001&sc=1000.

Colon, G., A. Gupta, and P. Mango. 1999. "M&A Malpractice." *McKinsey Quarterly* 1: 62–74.

Conklin, M. 1998. "Physicians' Dream Hits Rough Waters." *Rocky Mountain News*, September 6: 3G.

Connolly, C. 2008. "U.S. 'Not Getting What We Pay For.'" *Washington Post*, November 30, 2008. [Online article; retrieved 12/2/08.] www.washingtonpost.com/wp-dyn/content/story/2008/11/29/ST2008112902759.html.

Cook, S. W. 1984. "Cooperative Interaction in Multiethnic Contexts." In *Groups in Contact: The Psychology of Desegregation*, edited by N. Miller and M. B. Brewer, 155–85. Orlando, FL: Academic Press.

Cotton, K. 2008. "Fostering Intercultural Harmony in Schools: Research Findings." [Online article; retrieved 2/20/08.] www.nwrel.org/scpd/sirs/8/topsyn7.html.

Cutis, R. S. 2001. "Successful Collaboration Between Hospitals and Physicians: Process or Structure?" *Hospital Topics* 79 (2): 7–13.

Daft, R. L. 1998. *Organization Theory and Design.* Cincinnati, OH: South-Western College Publishing.

Davis, R. M. 2007. "Autonomy Versus Accountability: A Delicate Balance." *American Medical News* 50 (31). [Online article; retrieved 3/20/ 2008.] www.ama-assn.org/amednews/2007/08/20/edca0820.htm.

DeBoer, A., A. Iyenger, and T. Dudhela. 2008. "Beyond the Financial Rewards of Pay-for-Performance. [Online article; retrieved 1/30/08.] www.healthleadersmedia.com.

DerGurahian, J. 2008. "Docs Resist Staff Standard." *Modern Healthcare* 38 (25): 8–9.

Dickey, N. 2003. "Hospital–Physician Relations: A Response." *Frontiers of Health Services Management* 20 (2): 33–36.

Dubner, S. J., and S. D. Levitt. 2006. "Selling Soap." *New York Times*, September 24. [Online article; retrieved 9/10/08.] nytimes.com/2006/09/24/magazine/24wwln_freak.html.

Dukerich, J. M., B. R. Golden, and S. M. Shortell. 2002. "Beauty Is in the Eye of the Beholder: The Impact of Organizational Identification, Identity, and Image on the Cooperative Behaviors of Physicians." *Administrative Science Quarterly* 47 (3): 507–37.

Dynan L, G. J. Bazzoli, and L. R. Burns. 1998. "Assessing the Extent of Integration Achieved Through Physician–Hospital Arrangements." *Journal of Healthcare Management* 43 (3): 242–61.

Egger, E. 2001. "Market Memo: Developing Cost-Effective, Productive Physician Relations: Tips for Managing a Physician Clinic." *Health Care Strategic Management* 19 (1): 1–23.

Epperson, W., and P. Barakat. 2006. "'Us Versus Them' Struggle Continues Between Hospitals and Physicians." [Online article; retrieved 1/10/06]. www.acpe.org/click/archive/index.cfm?fuseaction=display&ID=13.

Evans, M. 2007. "CEOs Focus on Finance, Docs." *Modern Healthcare* 37 (1): 8–9.

Finger, A. L. 2000. "Happy Together: What Makes a Practice Endure?" *Medical Economics* 77 (9): 38.

Fiol, C. M. 1989. "A Semiotic Analysis of Corporate Language: Organizational Boundaries and Joint Venturing." *Administrative Science Quarterly* 34 (2): 277–303.

Fiol, C. M., M. G. Pratt, and E. J. O'Connor. 2009. "Managing Intractable Identity Conflicts." *Academy of Management Review* 34 (1): 32–55.

Firth-Cozens, J. 2004. "Organizational Trust: The Keystone to Patient Safety." *Quality and Safety in Healthcare* 13: 56–61.

Fisher E. S., D. O. Staiger, J. P. W. Bynum, and D. J. Gottlieb. 2006. "Creating Accountable Care Organizations: The Extended Hospital Medical Staff." *Health Affairs* 26 (1): 44–57.

Fisher, R. J. 1997. *Interactive Conflict Resolution*. Syracuse, NY: Syracuse University Press.

Fletcher, T. 2005. "The Impact of Physician Entrepreneurship on Escalating Health Care Costs." *Journal of the American College of Radiology* 2 (5): 411–14.

French, E. 2008. Personal communication, May 2.

Friedman, L. H. 2003. "Editorial." *Frontiers of Health Services Management* 20 (2): 1–2.

Fuhrmans, V. 2008. "Group Offers Doctors Bonuses for Better Care." *Wall Street Journal*, January 31: D4.

Gaertner, S. L., and J. F. Dovidio. 2000. *Reducing Intergroup Bias: The Common Ingroup Identity Model*. New York: Psychology Press.

Gaertner, S. L., J. F. Dovidio, J. A. Nier, C. M. Ward, and B. S. Banker. 1999. "Across Cultural Divides: The Value of a Superordinate Identity." In *Cultural Divides: Understanding and Overcoming Group Conflict*, edited by D. A. Prentice and D. T. Miller, 173–212. New York: Russell Sage Foundation.

Galbraith, J. R. 1973. *Designing Complex Organizations*. Reading, MA: Addison Wesley.

Gambetta, D. 1988. *Trust: Making and Breaking Cooperative Relations*. New York: Basil Blackwell.

Gillies R., H. Zuckerman, L. R. Burns, S. Shortell, J. Alexander, P. Budetti, and T. Waters. 2001. "Physician-System Relationships: Stumbling Blocks and Promising Practices." *Medical Care*, Suppl. 39 (71): 92–106.

Goldstein, S. M., and P. T. Ward. 2004. "Performance Effects of Physicians' Involvement in Hospital Strategic Decisions." *Journal of Service Research* 6 (4): 361–72.

Greene, J. 2000. "Physicians Enticed into Early Retirement: Frustrated by Managed Care Regulations and Bolstered by a Strong Market, Doctors Are Leaving the Bedside Earlier than Ever." [Online article; retrieved 2/21/06.] www.ama-assn.org/amednews/2000/07/24/prl20724.htm.

Gurin, P., T. Peng, G. Lopez, and B. A. Nagda. 1999. "Context, Identity, and Intergroup Relations." In *Cultural Divides: Understanding and Overcoming Group Conflict*, edited by D. A. Prentice and D. T. Miller, 133–70. New York: Russell Sage Foundation.

Guthrie, M., P. Froneberger, and D. Terry. 2005. *Survey of Better Performers in Cardiology*. Charlotte, NC: Premier, Inc.

Hagel, J., and J. S. Brown. 2005. "Productive Friction." *Harvard Business Review* (February): 83–91.

Haslam, S. A., and M. J. Platow. 2001. "The Link Between Leadership and Followership: How Affirming Social Identity Translates Vision into Action." *Personality and Social Psychology Bulletin* 27 (11): 1469–79.

Haslam, S. A., M. K. Ryan, T. Postmes, R. Spears, J. Jetten, and P. Webley. 2006. "Sticking to Our Guns: Social Identity as a Basis for the Maintenance of Commitment to Faltering Organizational Projects." *Journal of Organizational Behavior* 27 (6): 607–28.

Haugh, R. 2005. "Are You Looking for a Fresh Start with Your MDs?" [Online article; retrieved 11/03/08.] www.hhnmag.com/hhnmag_app/jsp/articledisplay.jsp?dcrpath=HHNMAG/PubsNewsArticle/data/0505HHN_InBox_Cover_Story&domain=HHNMAG.

Hekman, K. 2002. "If Only the Doctors Would Listen…to Administrators." [Online article; retrieved 2/11/06.] www.hekmangroup.com/articles/Article_IfOnlyDoctorsWoul dListen.pdf.

Herzig, M., and L. Chasin. 2006. *A Nuts and Bolts Guide from the Public Conversations Project.* Watertown, MA: Public Conversations Project.

———. 2004. *Allies or Adversaries: Revitalizing the Medical Staff Organization.* Chicago: Health Administration Press.

Holm, C. E. 2000. *Next Generation Physician–Health System Partnerships.* Chicago: Health Administration Press.

Hornsey, M., and M. Hogg. 2000a. "Assimilation and Diversity: An Integrative Model of Subgroup Relations." *Personality and Social Psychology Review* 4 (2): 143–56.

———. 2000b. "Subgroup Relations: A Comparison of Mutual Intergroup Differentiation and Common Ingroup Identity Models of Prejudice Reduction." *Personality and Social Psychology Bulletin* 26 (2): 242–56.

Hoskisson, R. E., and M. A. Hitt. 1994. *Downscoping.* New York: Oxford University Press.

Howard, C. 2003. "Restructuring Hospital–Physician Relationships for Future Success." *Frontiers of Health Services Management* 20 (2): 23–30.

Hubler, E. 1999. "Diagnosing Precedent's Downfall." *Denver Post,* July 4, I-01.

Hughes, J., and J. Weiss. 2007. "Simple Rules for Making Alliances Work." *Harvard Business Review* 85 (11): 1–10.

Hurley, R. 2006. "The Decision to Trust." *Harvard Business Review* (September): 55–62.

Jaklevic, C. 2001. "On Balance, a Positive Outcome." *Modern Healthcare* 31 (40): 36–40.

Jeter, J. 2003. Presentation at the University of Colorado Denver.

Jones, G. R. 2004. *Organizational Theory, Design, and Change.* Upper Saddle River, NJ: Prentice Hall.

Judge, W., and J. Ryman. 2001. "The Shared Leadership Challenge in Strategic Alliances: Lessons from the U.S. Health Care Industry." *Academy of Management Executive* 15 (2): 71–79.

Kaiser, L. 2000. Personal communication, October 22.

Kaufman, C. 1996. "Possible and Impossible Solutions to Ethnic and Civil Wars." *International Security* 20 (4): 135–75.

Kelman, H. C. 1998. "Interactive Problem Solving: An Approach to Conflict Resolution and its Application in the Middle East." *Political Science and Politics* 31 (2): 190–98.

———. 1997. "Group Processes in the Resolution of International Conflicts: Experiences from the Israeli–Palestinian Case." *American Psychologist* 52: 212–20.

———. 1983. "Conversations with Arafat: A Social-Psychological Assessment of the Prospects for Israeli-Palestinian Peace." *American Psychologist* 38: 208–16.

Kennedy, R. F. 1969. *Thirteen Days: A Memoir of the Cuban Missile Crisis.* New York: Norton.

Keohane, R. O., and J. S. Nye. 1977. *Power and Interdependence: World Politics in Transition.* Boston: Little, Brown.

Kertesz, L. 2004. "What Is Fueling the Increase in Health Care Costs: Mandates, Regulations, Litigation, Fraud, and Abuse Are Major Drivers." *Healthplan* 43 (3): 12–16.

Kilpatrick, R., and R. Leitch. 2004. "Teachers' and Pupils' Educational Experiences and School-Based Responses to the Conflict in Northern Ireland." *Journal of Social Issues* 60(3): 563–86.

Lambert, W. E., L. Mermigis, and D. M. Taylor. 1986. "Greek Canadians' Attitudes Towards Own Group and Other Canadian Ethnic Groups: A Test of the Multiculturalism Hypothesis." *Canadian Journal of Behavioral Science* 18(1): 35–51.

LeTourneau, B. 2004. "What Doctors Want." *Journal of Healthcare Management* 49 (4): 218–20.

Lord, J. D., and J. C. Catau. 1976. "School Desegregation, Busing, and Suburban Migration." *Urban Education* 10 (3): 275–94.

Lustig, I. 2002. "The Effects of Studying Distal Conflicts on the Perception of a Proximal One." Thesis, University of Haifa.

MacNulty, A., and J. Reich. 2008. "The Dynamic State of Physician–Hospital Alignment: Practical Strategies for Ensuring Your Success." ACPE member survey and interview results presentation, New York.

McGowan, R. A., and A. S. MacNulty. 2006. *Strategies for Strengthening Physician–Hospital Alignment.* Chicago: Society for Healthcare Strategy & Market Development.

Medical Group Management Association. 2008. "MGMA Cost Survey Reports: 2000–2006." *MGMA Connexion*, February 14.

Nerenz, D. 1992. "What Are the Essentials of System Integration?" *Frontiers of Health Services Management* 9: 58–61.

Norbut, M. 2003. "Physician Input Helps Hospital-Owned Group Make Money." [Online article; retrieved 10/06/08.] www.ama-assn.org/amednews/2003/04/07/bise0407.htm.

Northrup, T. 1989. "The Dynamic of Identity in Personal and Social Conflict." In *Intractable Conflicts and Their Transformation*, edited by L. Kriesberg, T. Northrup, and S. Thorson, 55–82. Syracuse, NY: Syracuse University Press.

O'Connor, E. J., and J. S. Bujak. 2001. "Trust, the Strategic Imperative: How to Successfully Build Physician–System Partnerships." *Healthcare Leadership and Management Report* (May): 6–9.

O'Connor, E. J., and C. M. Fiol. 2006. "Moving from Resistance to Support." *Physician Executive* 32 (5): 68–69.

———. 2002. "Diving into White Lightning." *MGMA Connexion* 2 (9): 22–24.

———. 1997. "Creating a Roadmap for Leading Change." In *Culture Shift: A Leader's Guide to Managing Change in Healthcare,* edited by J. Lowery, 39–60. Chicago: American Hospital Publishing.

O'Connor, E. J., C. M. Fiol, and M. Guthrie. 2006. "Separately Together: Build Unity by Strengthening Physician Groups." *Physician Executive* 32 (4): 16–21.

Osgood, C. E. 1962. *An Alternative to War and Surrender.* Champaign, IL: University of Illinois Press.

Pavia, L. 2003. "Becoming a 'Great Health Care Organization' to Weather the Next Industry Shakeout." *COR Healthcare Market Strategist.* [Online article; retrieved 1/12/04.] www.healthleadersmedia.com/content/49637/topic/ WS_HLM2_HOM/Becoming-a-Great-Healthcare-Organization-to-weather-the-next-industry-shakeout.html.

Performance Improvement Advisor. 2003. "Managers Can Take These Four Steps to Reduce Wasteful Work." *Performance Improvement Advisor* 76 (2): 162–63.

Porter, M. 2008. Personal communication, November 10.

Press Ganey. 2007. "Hospital Check-up Report: Physician Perspectives on American Hospitals." [Online article.] www.pressganey.com/galleries/default-file/physician-report.pdf.

Public Conversations Project. n.d. "Public Conversations." [Online article; retrieved 10/08/08.] www.publicconversations.org/pcp.

Reece, R. L. 2008. "The Physician Empowerment Movement." [Online article; retrieved 11/05/08.] www.healthleaders media.com/content/209307/topic/WS_HLM2_PHY/ The-Physician-Empowerment-Movement.html.

Reilly, P. 2004. "Off into the Sunset: Early Retirement of CEOs Poses Growing Problem." *Modern Healthcare* 14 (34): 8–9.

Robert, G. J. 1982. *Teaching Strategies for More Effective Integration*. Springfield, MA: Springfield Public Schools.

Rogers, E. M. 2003. *Diffusion of Innovations*, 5th ed. New York: Free Press.

Romano, M. 2004a. "Labor Unions Didn't Work: AMA Abandons Embattled In-House Group for Docs." *Modern Healthcare* 34 (22): 32–33.

———. 2004b. "Round 3: Doc Privileges Fight Heating Up: Lawsuit in Arkansas." *Modern Healthcare* 34 (7): 10–11.

Rundall, T. G. 2004. "Doctor–Manager Relationships in the United States and the United Kingdom." *Journal of Healthcare Management* 49 (4): 251–68.

Schlesinger, A. M. 1991. "Writing, and Rewriting, History." *New Leader* 74 (14): 12–14.

Semo, J. 2003. "Hospital–Medical Staff Relations: Strengthening Fragile Relationships." [Online article; retrieved 9/25/06.] www.asahq.org/Newsletters/2003/12-03/semo.html.

Shaman, H. 2007. "Improving Financial Health Through Quality Care." Presentation for the Patient Financial Services Subgroup of the Healthcare Financial Management Association. [Webcast.] www.hfma.org/forums/pfs/newsletter/PFSQIWinter2007.htm.

Sheehan, D. S., and M. Marcus. 1978. "Busing Status and Student Ethnicity: Effects on Student Achievement Scores." *Urban Education* 13 (1): 83–94.

Shortell, S. 1991. *Effective Hospital–Physician Relationships.* Chicago: Health Administration Press.

Silversin, J., and M. J. Kornacki. 2000. "Creating a Physician Compact That Drives Group Success." *MGM Journal* 47 (3): 54–62.

Smith, M. 2002. "Success Rates for Different Types of Organizational Change." *Performance Improvement* 41 (1): 26–33.

Strode, R. 2004. "Hospital–Physician Joint Ventures: Threat or Opportunity?" *Healthcare Financial Management* 58 (7): 80–86.

Stubblefield, A. 2005. *The Baptist Healthcare Journey to Excellence: Creating a Culture That WOWs!* Hoboken, NJ: John Wiley & Sons.

Svejenova, S. 2006. "How Much Does Trust Really Matter? Some Reflections on the Significance and Implications of Madhok's Trust-Based Approach." *Journal of International Business Studies* 37: 12–20.

Tamari, S. 2002. "How Narratives of the Naqba Have Evolved in the Memories of Exiled Palestinians." *Journal of Politics, Economics, and Culture* 9 (4): 101–9.

Thomas, K. W., and W. H. Schmidt. 1976. "A Survey of Managerial Interests with Respect to Conflict." *Academy of Management Journal* (June): 317.

Trapp, D. 2007. "Health Insurance Premiums up 6.1%, Fast Outpacing Inflation and Wages." *American Medical News*, October 1. [Online information.] www.amaassn.org/amednews/2007/10/01/ gvl11001.htm

Troebst, S. 1998. "Conflict in Kosovo: Failures of Prevention? An Analytical Documentation, 1989–1998." Working Paper 1. Flensburg, Germany: European Centre for Minority Issues.

Tyler, T. R., and S. Blader. 2000. *Co-operation in Groups: Procedural Justice, Social Identity and Behavioral Engagement.* Philadelphia, PA: Psychology Press.

Weber, D. 2006. "Friction Points!" *Physician Executive* 32 (4): 6–11.

Weiss, J., and J. Hughes. 2005. "Want Collaboration? Accept—and Actively Manage—Conflict." *Harvard Business Review* (March): 93–101.

Weymier, R. E. 2004. "The Hospital/Physician Divide: Understanding the Drivers of Their Relationships." *Physician Executive* 30 (3): 60–62.

Wilensky, R. G., N. Wolter, and M. M. Fischer. 2007. "Gain Sharing: A Good Concept Getting a Bad Name?" *Health Affairs* 26 (1): w58–w67.

Wilper, A. P., S. Woolhandler, K. E. Lasser, D. McCormick, S. L. Cutrona, D. H. Bor, and D. U. Himmelstein. 2008. "Waits to See an Emergency Department Physician: U.S. Trends and Predictors, 1997–2004." *Health Affairs* 27 (2): 84–95.

Wolf, R. L., and R. J. Simon. 1975. "Does Busing Improve the Racial Interactions of Children?" *Educational Researcher* 4 (1): 5–10.

Wong, E. 2002. "Bankruptcy Hint by United Airlines." *New York Times*, August 15, A1.

Zhang, J. 2007. "Growth in U.S. Health-Care Spending Slows Again." *Wall Street Journal: Eastern Edition* 249 (7): A2.

Index

'Abrasiveness, creative,' 149–151,
  165–166
Accountability
  of physicians and hospitals, 18
  effect of negative connections on,
    87
  relationship to autonomy, 149
Administrative departments, hierarchical structure of, 115,
  124
Administrator leaders, 124
Administrators
  beliefs about physicians, 173
  challenges facing, 8
  'collective' culture of, 28, 31–32
  commonalties among, 118–119
  division of labor among,
    115–116
  as fragmented group, 112–113
  group mobilization of, 116–117
  interdependence with physicians,
    140–141
  lack of group identification, 113

networking among, 117–118
  as PAR Process transition team
    leaders, 61–62
  performance measurement of,
    121
Advisory Board, 35
Albanian-Serbian conflict, 96–97
Alliances
  corporate, 125, 126
  strategic, 20–23
American College of Healthcare
  Executives (ACHE), 4,
  117–118
American Hospital Association
  (AHA), 21, 22, 25–26
American Medical Association
  (AMA)
  failed unionization initiative of,
    123
  statement on freedom in medical
    practice, 149
Apple Computer, 32–33, 49
Arab-Israeli conflict, 88, 97, 98, 151

Arafat, Yassar, 97
Ashtabula County Medical Center, 22
Autonomy, of physicians and administrators, 49–50, 116
associated with separate togetherness, 57–58
as barrier to hospital-physician relations, 71
relationship to accountability, 149

Baptist Health Care, Pensacola, Florida, 122
Behavioral strategies, for separate togetherness development, 147–148
Beth Israel Deaconess Medical Center, Cardiovascular Institute, 122
Bias, intergroup, 40
Blue Cross and Blue Shield, 151
Bonding, between administrators and physicians, 33–34. *See also* Separate group security
Boston University, 6
Boundaries
reinforcement of, 148
softening of, 148–149
Bressanelli, Leo, 143
Brideau, Leo, 3
Brigham and Women's Hospital, 122
Buffering strategies, 76–77
Buffers, neutral, 173–174
Built to Last (Collins and Porras), 32–33
Bujak, Joseph, 51
Inside the Physician Mind, 116

Business models, of healthcare delivery, 17, 18

Canadians, separate togetherness of, 148
Cedars-Sinai Medical Center, 154
Center for Health Futures, 141
Center for Studying Health System Change, 8
Cesarean deliveries, unnecessary, 7
Change
failed attempts for, 71
readiness for. *See also* Phase One of PAR Process
resistance to, 70–77
risk reduction approach to, 71–72, 75–77
shared gain approach to, 71, 74–75;
shared pain approach to, 71, 72–74
Chief executive officers (CEOs)
attitudes toward retreats, 33–34
beliefs about physicians, 35
early retirement of, 8
ratings of physician-administrator relations by, 59
Churchill, Winston, 169, 179
Citizenship behaviors, 113
Clinical practice guidelines, non-adherence to, 7
Clinton, Bill, 7
Codes of conduct, 11–12
Colie, Russell, 124
Collaboration
failed approaches to, 48
fusion approach to 143
graduated reciprocation approach to, 95–96

in hospital-owned physician practices, 180

relationship to conflict, 150

separate group security-based, 112

separate togetherness-based, 50–51

in specialty treatment, 122

Columbia St. Mary's hospital system, 3

Commitment

effect of separate group security on, 113–114

to improved hospital-physician relations, 69–70

Commonalties, intergroup, 139

identification of, 118–119

Communication

open, 36, 37

poor, as conflict cause, 36

role in separate togetherness, 147, 164

role in trust, 36, 37

Community Memorial Hospital, Ventura, California, 11–12

Compacts

definition of, 145

rewriting of, 145–146, 162–164, 179

sponsors' support for, 153–154

Compensation. *See also* Income for PAR Process involvement, 77

Competition, hospital-physician

case study of, 9–11

effect of structural integration on, 19–20

Conduct, codes of, 11–12

Conflict, 3-16. *See also* Ethnic conflicts

as basis for healthcare system's failure, 10

as 'creative abrasiveness,' 149–151

as group's defining characteristic, 52

healthcare costs-related, 4, 5–6

negative consequences of, 70, 73–74

relationship to collaboration, 150

risk reduction approach to, 71–72, 75–77

shared gain approach to, 71, 74–75

shared pain approach to, 71, 72–74

worldview differences-related, 28, 31–32

Conflicts of interest, among stakeholders, 70–71

Conflicts-of-interest policies, 11–12

Conflict transformation, 90–91

Cooking, fusion, 142–143

Corporate alliances, 125, 126

Corporate executives, lack of trust in, 75

Corporatization, of healthcare, 8–9

Cosi Fan Tutte (Mozart), 96

Cost-containment efforts, 141

Cost-plus reimbursement, 17

Covenant Healthcare, 144

'Creative abrasiveness,' 149–151, 165–166

Credentialing, hospitals' withholding of, 20

Credibility

communication strategies component, 147, 164, 179

components of, 141–152

creative abrasiveness component, 149–151, 165–166

dissemination of, 154–155

exercises for promotion of, 161–166

failure of, 178–179

fusion approach component, 142–143, 146

importance of, 140–141

integrating mechanisms approach in, 144–145

leadership for, 60

overcoming resistance to, 140, 153–154, 161

purpose of, 139, 178

purpose statement component, 142–144, 153, 161–162, 179

reasons for resistance to, 152–153

reinforcement in, 151–152

rewriting of compacts component, 145–146, 162–164, 179

self-assessment exercises of, 157–160

softening of boundaries component, 148–149, 165

Physician(s)

beliefs about administrators, 173

beliefs about hospital CEOs, 35

challenges facing, 8–9

commonalties among, 118–119

early retirement of, 8–9

expert culture of, 28, 31–32

as fragmented group, 113

group mobilization of, 116–117

interdependence with administrators, 140–141

lack of group identification, 113

motivations of, 114

negative attitudes toward medical practice, 8–9

networking among, 117

performance measurement of, 121–122

subgroups of, 116

as transition team leaders, 61–62

younger, 12, 35

Physician Administration Relations Process. *See* PAR (Physician Administration Relations) Process

Physician employment models, 25

Physician executives, clinical *versus* administrative concerns of, 124

Physician-hospital organizations (PHOs), 21–22, 23

failure of, 25

Physician leaders

attitudes toward retreats, 33–34

ratings of physician-administrator relations by, 59

role in PAR Process, 60–61

role in performance management system development, 121

Physician loyalty teams, 122

Physician practices

in competition with hospitals, 11

hospitals' acquisition of, 19, 25, 180

Physicians Interactive, 117

Porter, Michael, 4

Precedent Health Care, Denver,

Verispan, Ten 100 Integrated
Health Networks report, 144
Vertical integration, of hospital–physician relations, 18–19
Vigilance, 181
Vision-based approach, to hospital–physician relations, 31–43
effect of distrust on, 35–37,
38–39, 40
failure of, 34–35, 39–41, 49
identification of commonalties
for, 118–119
limitations of, 170
rationale for, 32–33

role of open communication in,
36, 37
role of trust in, 35–37
separate togetherness-based success of, 180
Vulnerability
in information sharing, 179–180
in interdependence, 139

Web sites, use for networking, 117
Welch, Jack, 33, 40–41, 169, 170
Worldviews
conflicting, 28, 31–32, 36
consistency among, 89–90

About the Authors

C. Marlena Fiol, MBA, PhD, has more than 30 years of experience in strategic management and organizational design. She has worked with hospital administrators, board members, and physician leaders to identify their core competencies, clarify market demands, develop strategic directions, and implement the tactics required to compete successfully in changing markets. As a transition specialist, she has worked with healthcare organizations to identify stakeholder positions, develop leadership skills, and design the organizational structures and reporting relationships needed to effectively implement high-quality delivery systems.

Dr. Fiol is a professor of strategy and health administration at the University of Colorado–Denver and a principal with the Implementation Institute, a Denver-based consulting and training firm that specializes in clarifying strategic directions and removing barriers to their successful implementation. She has authored numerous research articles, book chapters, and papers on topics related to physician–hospital relations, strategic thinking, organizational learning, and change management. Her previous book with Ed O'Connor, *Reclaiming Your Future: Entrepreneurial Thinking in Health Care*, provides practical ideas and examples for healthcare leaders who are committed to being the architects of their own futures.

Dr. Fiol holds an MBA and a PhD in strategic management from the University of Illinois at Urbana-Champaign. In addition to her teaching, research, and consulting activities, Dr. Fiol has been a frequent speaker at international, national, and regional meetings. She can be reached at (303) 573-1273 or by e-mail at marlena. fiol@ucdenver.edu.

Edward J. O'Connor, MBA, PhD, is a Professor of Management and Health Administration at the University of Colorado–Denver, a Principal with the Implementation Institute, and a faculty member of the American College of Physician Executives. He is also a member of the American College of Healthcare Executives and Medical Group Management Association. As the author of more than 150 research articles, book chapters, papers, and technical documents, Dr. O'Connor's work focuses on physician–hospital relations, change management, visionary strategic leadership, conflict resolution, and entrepreneurship. His prior book with Marlena Fiol, *Reclaiming Your Future: Entrepreneurial Thinking in Health Care*, provides practical ideas and examples for healthcare leaders who are committed to being the architects of their own futures.

In addition to holding management positions with General Electric and providing consulting services for hospitals, health systems, and group practices, Dr. O'Connor has personally engaged in several entrepreneurial business ventures. He holds an MBA from the Harvard Business School and a PhD in industrial/organizational psychology from the University of Akron. He has previously served on business and psychology faculties at the Universities of Georgia, Tennessee, and Texas and at the Georgia Institute of Technology.

Dr. O'Connor is a frequent keynote speaker at national and regional healthcare meetings and is known for his dynamic, high-energy style. He can be reached at (303) 573-1273 or by e-mail at edward.oconnor@ucdenver.edu.